". . . *the* herbal that we've needed for a long time."

David Copperfield
Well-Being Magazine

". . . the most clear and readable herbal I've found. Because of his extremely practical and down-to-earth descriptions, the author makes herbs more accessible to lay people than ever before. This is an important contribution in an era when individuals are demanding more control over their health and more holistic methods of healing."

Barbara Clutter, M.D.
Women's Health Services
Santa Fe

". . . an invaluable reference for the ethnobotanist, anthropologist, pharmacognosist, and, indeed, anyone interested in one of the rich traditions of medicine."

George Conway
School of Medicine
University of New Mexico

Medicinal Plants

OF THE
MOUNTAIN
WEST

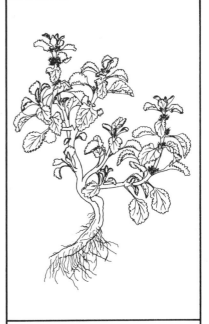

Michael Moore

A guide
to the identification,
preparation, and uses of
traditional medicinal
plants found in the
mountains, foothills,
and upland areas of the
American West.

MUSEUM OF NEW MEXICO PRESS

The publication of this book was made possible by a grant from the Museum of New Mexico Foundation.

10 9 8

Printed in the United States of America.

ISBN: 0-89013-104-X (paperbound) 0-89013-107-4 (clothbound)
Library of Congress Catalog Card Number: 79-620000

The drawings in this book are by Nora Ausubel, Phyllis Hughes, and Y. Matsumura (from Edible Native Plants of the Rocky Mountains, *by H. D. Harrington, published by the University of New Mexico Press), and from sources including the Southwest Parks and Monuments Association and the University of California Press. Left-hand cover photo courtesy New Mexico Commerce and Industry Department. Color section photographs by Philip L. Carter, Susan Hill, Tom Duckworth, Sharon Wirtz, and the University of New Mexico Herbarium. Graphic production by Rachel Abrams.*

Although every effort has been made to insure accuracy and reliability, the publisher assumes no responsibility for the effects of the techniques described herein for the preparation and use of these traditional medicinal plants.

FOREWORD

Michael Moore has written *the* herbal that we've needed for a long time. As publisher of *Well-Being Magazine,* a journal extensively concerned with herbs, I have been frustrated by herbals that copy their information from earlier books or are incomplete in scope. In this regard Michael Moore has spared us—and waited twelve years before sharing his wealth of mosly firsthand experience. And the information is here: little known effects, exact dosages, and estimates of relative reliability make this book extremely valuable. Add to this the information on the herbs' active ingredients, indications of toxicity, the exacting descriptions of the plants, the habitats, and harvesting instructions and you have a book that is of great value to herb lovers, practitioners, and scientists.

The author is a curious combination of trader, herbalist, pharmacologist, gatherer, botanist, physician, gardener, teacher, folk historian . . . in short, a rennaissance man when it comes to herbs. It was actually Michael Moore who first taught me about herbs and who unknowingly led me toward becoming the publisher of a natural health care magazine. That, of course, is a long story but suffice it to say that the simple and potent style with which he shared his information never left me. And I believe that what he has shared in this herbal will have an even greater impact on your future involvement with herbs.

One last thing. I believe this book will raise herbalism to a new level of credibility. Too many folk tales and not enough hard twentieth century data have given herbs an undeservedly unscientific image. The fact is that herbs are worthy of a place in today's medical pharmacy. Moore puts it all in perspective when he states that herbs should fill the void between health and acute disease, a void that occurred because of the medical profession's romance with "miracle drugs" like penicillin. This herbal is filled with the solid information that will go a long way toward filling that void. Thank you, Michael Moore.

David Copperfield, Publisher
Well-Being Magazine
Santa Cruz, California
November 1978

ACKNOWLEDGEMENTS

I would like to acknowledge the encouragement, constructive skepticism, and/or technical assistance of the following individuals: Greg Gorman, M.D., Richard Moskowitz, M.D., Dr. William Martin, Paul Hummel, D.C., Noreen Sullivan, D.C., Jay Scherer, N.D., Scott Gershen, N.D., William Lesessier, N.D., Gail Tierney, Martha Baca and the intrepid George Conway. None of them should be held responsible for the book; they just threw pieces of information and insights into my cerebral cauldron . . . some of them may not recognize the final product. I would like to thank Richard Polese and Jim Mafchir of the Museum of New Mexico for their genial doggedness; without them I would still be working on this book . . . also for her delicate insistence, my editor, Sarah Nestor. I should also mention my old herb cronies from Topanga, Michael and John, and my parents for their patience and time.

This book is dedicated to the women: Velia, Michele, and Chavela.

Michael Moore
Santa Fe
December, 1978

CONTENTS

8

INTRODUCTION

This book can fit no set categories, since it is, by intent, generalist. It isn't strictly a botanical text, field guide, herb book, or medical treatise; neither is it a textbook on ethnobotany, pharmacognosy, or folk remedies. Rather, it is a bit of all of these. During my twelve years of active interest in herbal medicine and my ten years as a merchant, picker, and teacher, I have had to learn some small or large part of all these fields in order to better understand and use botanical medicines. As it is my livelihood, I have had time to assemble a lot of this varying nonsense into a reasonably coherent package so that others, with their own livelihoods and interests, may be able to make use of my synthesis. Many may wish to use this book as a basic reference source for home remedies, both in their own gathering and, when plants are out of season or unavailable, in purchasing. Others, such as physicians, pharmacists, chiropractors, nurses, and therapists, can find it a useful starting point for further endeavors.

I have picked all the plants in this book in the wild, and their uses and dosages are the result of firsthand or reliable secondhand information filtered through my own preferences and opinions. The book is full of opinions, and the reader is encouraged to view them with a jaundiced eye. It is at least based primarily on personal experience and not, as is sometimes the case in recent herb books, on gleanings from the bone piles of older texts.

One thing that has always bothered me about many herb books is a chronic pussyfooting in regards to dosage and qualitative opinions. Another complaint of mine is their proclivity to treat herbs as sacrosanct, wholistic entities, divorced from and above medical and pharmaceutical practices. In fact, over half of the generas in this book have been official drug plants at various times in the *United States Pharmacopeia* or the *National Formulary*. It is only the changing therapies, dogmas, and habits of the medical professions that have resulted in the "crazy-uncle-in-the-attic" attitude towards galenic and herbal medicines.

Above all, there is a need for some general material on medicinal plants of the West. During the eighteenth and nineteenth centuries when the main settling of land east of the Rockies was accomplished, herbs were the major part of the armamentarium of the physician, and Indian medicine was still intact enough to serve as raw material for pharmaceutical evaluation. On the other hand the West was settled largely in the twentieth century, at a time when medicine was turning away from plants as major drug sources, and the native Indian populations, decimated and isolated, were losing touch with their traditional paths. The many Spanish-speaking peoples of the Southwest, along with their herbal traditions, were largely ignored, with the result that this rich lode of empirical lore has been seldom utilized by the population at large. (The few exceptions are central and northern New Mexico, southern California, and southern Texas, where there are large concentrations of Spanish-speaking people.) The result of this is the present state of what passes for American herb usage, in which ninety percent of the plants are native to the eastern third of the United States. The only herbs from the West with any substantial herb use in most of the country are Cascara Sagrada, Yerba Santa, and Chaparral (Larrea).

Herbal remedies represent far more than a wholistic fad or a total rejection of traditional medicine. They help to fill the overwhelming void between health and acute disease, a void left when the medical profession discovered penicillin and began its romance with the concept of "miracle drugs." I have known perfectly intelligent physicians whose sole regularly used reference manuals were the *Physicians' Desk Reference* and Goodman & Gillman, both drug manuals. Their patients have come to expect, and receive, prescriptions as their only therapy. At best doctors might have had a year of pharmacology in medical school (probably six months); the actual experts on drugs and their interactions, however, are the pharmacists who count out the pills. Yet how many doctors ever ask a pharmacist for advice? Very few, I imagine.

Drugs can save lives in serious, acute diseases and may alleviate or even cure some chronic problems, but they are very poorly suited for the vast majority of chronic and minor ailments. With their many and not-so-subtle side effects they often hinder the innate ability of the organism to heal itself. Iatrogenic (drug caused) diseases affect most Americans at one time or another, yet a man or woman has innate disease defenses of incredible complexity, far surpassing the totality of all drug therapies. A disease that has run its course, with the body's being allowed to heal itself in its own fashion and chronology, is far less likely to return as a chronic ailment. With many patients seeking a pill and a pat on the back for self-limiting disorders and often unwilling to accept responsibility for their own healing, overworked physicians will prescribe drugs as a knee-jerk therapy, often circumventing and interfering with the body's responses. This may allow the imbalance to occur at a later date, as the full cycle of defenses has been prevented, until the imbalance sets in as an ingrained habit called chronic disease. Although the life span has been greatly increased in the last hundred years, this is not generally the result of drugs but of preventative medicine and sanitation. We no longer defecate in our water supplies and we wash our hands before delivering babies. The more virulent microorganisms that can penetrate the defenses of healthy individuals have been systematically controlled . . . at least in the industrialized world. What remains is a miasma of degeneracy diseases — the final states of the chronic imbalances, diseases that drug therapy and surgery have been singularly unable to deal with.

In contrast to the single-mindedness of drugs, the biochemical compositions of plants are varying, complex, and subtle. This generally makes them inappropriate for the chronic disease that becomes acute or for a seriously flawed defense system. At the same time, they are composed of fairly predictable groups of substances that our bodies have long since evolved methods of dealing with. In fact the very act of excreting some plant substances is often their mode of effect, since they are usually of little use as food or building materials. These predictable means of excretion explain why some herbs act to stimulate urine production, sweat and sebaceous secretions, lymph flow, and liver function.

The herbs in this book will often supply palliative relief (sedative, laxative, etc.) like many drugs, but they will do this without interfering with normal healing processes or having the residual toxicities of many drugs. Others will react in an opposite fashion, acting to stimulate and even temporarily aggravate the healing processes of the body. The concept of stimulating a fever seems to run counter to much accepted medical tradition, but when a fever is viewed as the only appropriate defense response at that stage of an infection, and when such an herb will also increase sweating which brings heat outward as well as cooling the skin by evaporation and speeding excretion of waste products, this approach seems more rational than suppressing the fever with salicylates. In fact, many "diseases" and

10

their symptoms are in reality perfectly appropriate body defense responses and should not be depressed at all. A simple inflammation is the reaction of the tissues to an infection or irritation, and results in quicker tissue repair or the isolation of the invader. Instead of lessening the inflammation through anti-inflammatories, it would be more sensible to stimulate it through rubifacients, moist heat, and a systemic vasodilator such as Bayberry, ginger, or capsicum.

This stimulation of defense responses, termed a *healing crisis* in naturopathic medicine, is the cornerstone of most alternative healing therapies, although herbs are only one way to bring it about. Plants that stimulate such responses are termed *alteratives* in herbal practice.

In such a use of an herb, however, there is the presumption that the person is in basic good health with reasonably attuned and appropriate defense mechanisms. They should be used with much caution for young children, the elderly, and individuals with chronic poor health or serious hereditary imbalances, as such people may overreact. In any case, common sense should be used when a defense reaction seems excessive—the body is not always correct in its assessment of the problem, or in the magnitude of its response. There are no fixed methods to apply to the human predicament, there is no single all-pervasive rule to follow, since medicine is not a science but an art. The therapies or uses recommended in this book cannot be treated as Holy Writ; they are simply sensible guidelines and majority effects.

The herbs I discuss will have no beneficial effects at all for some people — nothing works for everybody. Such factors as race, diet, sex, and even the time of day have many and complex effects that are poorly understood or even ignored, and the ingestion of biochemical substances to promote healing is only a small part of the whole.

Certainly herbs alone cannot bring relief to individuals whose very life style may be the cause of their illness. A person who has gradually developed a gastric ulcer and insists on coffee and doughnuts for breakfast, a ham sandwich and beer for lunch, a sullen stress-filled dinner, and endless rehashings of daily traumas and frustrations while sleeping cannot obtain more than the slightest relief from Barberry Root or Hound's Tongue. That is beyond the help of a mere herbal tea and beyond the scope of this book.

The avowed function of any healing therapy should be to enable the organism to heal itself by strengthening its defenses or, failing that, to caulk the cracks. The ways are legion, from the various biochemical approaches (allopathic, homeopathic, and herbal medicines) to naturopathy, chiropractice, rolfing, polarity therapy, meditation, rebirth, organized religions, faith healing, etc. The native and naturalized plants I have listed are a valid part of this healing circle.

If you like lists, here is one to keep in mind when using this book:

1. Be sure of the plant you are picking.
2. If the herb makes you sick, take less or throw it away.
3. If it doesn't work, use more or forget it entirely.
4. Trust your own judgment above all.
5. That which stimulates can irritate; that which helps can hurt.
6. If you don't get better or get worse quickly, call your doctor.

11

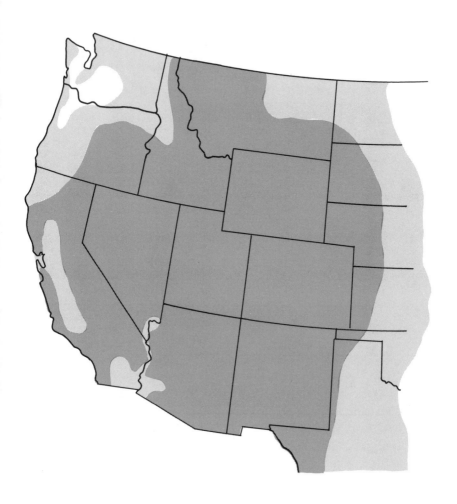

The plants described in this book can be found in the mountains, foothills, and upland areas in the regions encompassed by the shading on this map.

Dark shading — Primary area covered by this book.
Light shading — Where one may also expect to find many of the plants included in this book.

FORMAT EXPLANATION

COMMON NAME: Here I have listed many "unofficial" plants, having found their functions similar to or greater than those of "official" plants. Some purists may complain that I have used a name improperly when applying it to related but unknown plants. That Arnica was first introduced as a remedy in Europe is as much accidental as anything else, and the fact that *Arnica montana* is listed as the official species is more a matter of our predominantly European heritage than of any preeminant value that particular species has. Official species names are often little more than type guides. Pennyroyal of commerce may be one of several species common to the United States, yet they are all lumped together as *Hedeoma pulegioides*. Gentian species all have a very similar pharmacology, yet people have trundled off to pharmacies (then) and herb stores (now) for centuries in the United States to buy roots dug in the Pyrenees of Europe.

I have tried to retain the most common name used in the West when the herb is addressed as a medicinal plant. A plant with a Spanish name such as Inmortal may be listed in field guides as spider milkweed, but its only remedy use comes from the Hispanics in Arizona, New Mexico, and southern Colorado. Although Poleo grows in many parts of North America and has always been used by a few individuals, its only consistent place is in New Mexico, where it bears that name.

Unfortunately, it is impractical to include the many Indian names for plants in this book. Phonetic renderings are highly variable; some tribes may adapt the name from another tribe or use the Spanish name, or, as in Oshá, have dozens of different names, all meaning "Bear Medicine." Besides, most Indians know at least some of their native medicines . . . the rest of us usually don't. For clarification, the common names of plants discussed in the text are capitalized.

LATIN NAME: Although the original intent of Latin naming was to create a universal, inviolate nomenclature, that is hardly the case any more. I have tried to list the most commonly used species names from the plant manuals of the West or, where two names are equally employed, to list both. For those unfamiliar with Latin names, the first name is the genera (like Chavez); the second name is the species (like Maria); the last name is the "Natural Order" or the superfamily it is found in (like "Spanish-speaking New Mexican").

OTHER NAMES: These include some of the more common English or Spanish names that are encountered, as well as some of the more frequent alternate Latin names.

DESCRIPTION: The ideal circumstance is to go into the field with an experienced person. Most universities, junior colleges, and herbariums have classes or conducted plant walks, as well as extension and adult education programs. If you have never attempted to identify plants from manuals, even as unorthodox a manual as this one, it is always better to break the ice in such a manner. There are native plant societies in many areas as well as many individuals in the West that give herb walks.

Lacking such resources, or having some background other than strict botany, you will have little difficulty with the plant descriptions in this book, since the botanical jargon has been kept to a minimum. If you have training in botany you will probably tear your hair out, as there are instances where thirty words have been necessary to describe a plant detail when one technical word would have sufficed.

13

In general, where there are a number of similar species I have tried to include the predominant characteristics of the whole group, emphasizing distinctive peculiarities—those most likely to be noticed. The growing conditions and local varieties may greatly alter certain gross aspects, such as height, density of foliage, color of leaf or flower, scent, and the like. The illustrations are as typical of the overall appearance as possible, but many plants have the infuriating habit of adapting to their locality and not to this book. Remember that some plants maintain a uniform appearance wherever they are found, while others change subtly from meadow to meadow. In the Willow family (Salicaceae), Poplars maintain this uniformity, with Aspens never changing appearance from Alaska to Mexico, Pacific to Atlantic. The species, subspecies, and varieties of Willows, however, number well into the hundreds, with many local adaptations having characteristics of several types. A "species," therefore, as well as a genera, is often only an approximation, a series of fine lines arbitrarily dividing similar plants. With fewer plants and more botanists, certain groups of adaptive plants are fair game for master and doctoral "review." It is the accumulated weight of these "clarifications" that can cause the plethora of Latin names for the same plant.

HABITAT: This has to be approximate, since distribution of plants, their relationship to each other and our species, and distinct changes in plant ecologies from year to year make it impossible to define absolutely. A few of the introduced plants, particularly those with barbed seeds, can be expected almost anywhere. Habitats listed bear only approximate likeness to actual conditions, as I have taken into consideration the fact that most people will not venture much more than a quarter of a mile off a road looking for plants. The two-legged mountain goat and horse packer may encounter plants far removed from their supposed habitat. For the rest of us, logging roads and hiking trails are sufficient to get us up and away from the resort towns. The many herbariums in the West, usually at universities and botanical gardens, are an excellent beginning in locating plants of a more obscure nature. Listings of more than twenty years past can be very misleading, however, since a stand of Angelica that was listed as abundant in the folder (collected 1936) may, once you get there, be a ski condominium with electrified barbed wire and moat. Remember, also, that altitudes will vary, depending on whether the plant is in moister Pacific mountains (lower altitudes) or the inland ranges (higher altitudes). A plant found at 7,000 feet in New Mexico may be found at 5,000 feet in Montana. Plants descend to lower altitudes the further north they grow.

COLLECTING: Make a point of picking only plants growing in prime locations. Individuals with many insect holes and obvious poor health are probably located at the extremes of their preferred growing conditions and may also have distinctly atypical biochemistries. Always check around after you have located a needed plant. There may be a whole field of it over the next rise or around the bend in the road. On the other hand, they may be the only two plants in the whole valley—and should be left alone. Furthermore, a plant common in one state may be an endangered or protected plant in another, so check first, if in doubt.

Certain conservation practices are always necessary. If a plant grows in large stands, never pick more than a third of the plants. If it is a larger, solitary bush or tree, never pick more than a third of the foliage or twigs and preferably from the borders of the plant, leaving the older central growth to regenerate outwards. If you are digging roots, dig no more than half of the immediately visible plants and the largest of the group, leaving the younger to grow and reseed. Fill up your holes if

14

they are deep; a meadow full of potholes is an invitation to erosion. The mountain forest may seem omnipotent, but it is frequently a delicately balanced ecology, easily thrown off. When bark is needed, check the trees after a good rainstorm; there may be large, newly fallen limbs with fresh bark. Otherwise, choose older limbs with only a few leaves at the tips and remove the whole limb before stripping the bark.

COLLECTING METHODS:

Method A: This is basically for aboveground foliage that forms distinct stems. The stems are cut below the lowest green leaves and bundled, facing the same direction, then bound one or two inches from the cut ends with #31, 32, or 33 rubber bands (one-eighth inch wide). Twine or wrapped wire may be used but can allow pieces to drop as they shrink and dry. For moist herbs such as Mint or Horsetail, bundles should never exceed, at the tied end, the outside diameter of the neck of a beer bottle. Drier herbs of a bulky nature, such as Mormon Tea, may be tied in larger bundles without fear of the inner branches mildewing or molding. If the plants are dirty or very hairy they may be washed under cool water, squeezed gently, rinsed, shaken of excess water, and hung to dry. Washed bundles must be smaller to prevent spoilage. In reality, very few herbs need to be washed if they are picked away from the roadsides. This is always better anyway, as many herbs absorb exhaust substances when directly roadside.

Herbs should *never* be dried in sunlight; instead, hung from hooks or nails in shaded areas with adequate circulation. They should be hung until both the top and bottom of the herbs are brittle-dry. After drying they may be stored in a variety of ways, but they are usually cut first. For most herbs in blossom, the flowering half of the bundle is chopped into regular half-inch to one-inch segments with rose shears or kitchen scissors. The remaining half of the stems are stripped of leaves and the bare stems discarded. When the stems are small or weak, as in Cleavers, Pennyroyal, or Poleo, the complete bundle should be cut and used.

Canning jars and cleaned reused jars with tops are the optimum storage containers. Be sure to label the contents and, if you have suppressed Virgo tendencies, you might even methodically label the date and picking location for future reference. Coffee cans or even plastic bags are also appropriate, but paper bags should not be used. Storage should be in a cool, dark area. If your area or house has grain weavils (little brown nasties that live in dried flour bins), then a pinch of diatomaceous earth should be added to the herbs and dispersed by shaking. This is a problem in moderate and high-humidity areas, particularly in stored roots and flowers. Most freshly picked, coarsely chopped herbs will last a year at full strength. After two years they should be discarded.

Method B: For large roots. If they are aromatic, as Angelica or Oshá, they should be split once or twice from top to bottom and dried loosely in a shallow box or on newspapers. This prevents exposing much of the oil cells to the air and evaporation. Nonaromatic roots may simply be cut sideways and laid loosely until dry. Cross sections should be no more than one-fourth inch thick. They may be cut smaller still after dried and lightly chopped even further for tea or encapsulating with a grain mill or blender. Most finer processing should only take place before actual use, since large root sections can stay potent for years.

Method C: This is for moist, highly perishable herbs, either flowers, fruits, or small damp plants and roots. Also the ideal drying method for any thinly sliced fruit or vegetable. A length of cheesecloth at least twenty-four inches wide is stapled or tacked along its front width to a ceiling or the underside of a wall cabinet in a well ventilated area. A sag in the cloth of eight or ten inches should be allowed, then staple or tack again about two feet away and repeat as long as the cloth or available ceiling or cabinet area allows. The draped cloth between the tacking allows for the loose placement of the herbs in the panels. These should be patted periodically from underneath to redistribute and speed drying. Another method for smaller quantities is an open-topped box covered with cheesecloth. In extremities newspaper can be used if the herbs are loosely laid. Store as in Method A.

Method D: For tree barks. The branch or tree should be still fresh. Make shallow cuts around the diameter every foot or two and length-cuts every two or three inches. The strips should be pulled off the inner wood and threaded on coarse thread, wire, or a straightened, oiled coat hanger. (The oil prevents rust.) Hang the bark strips in well ventilated shade until dry, then chop or break into smaller pieces for storing.

MEDICINAL USE: Several considerations must be kept in mind when using herbs to remedy a physical imbalance or disease. Acute illnesses, those with quick onset, strong symptoms, and a self-limiting nature, should be treated simply, using one or two herbs. The purpose of botanicals here is to give comfort, speed defense reactions, and limit and define the course to prevent complications or prolonging. Common sense is paramount, since the remedies may not be sufficient or may cause an overreaction. The use of salicylate herbs (Birch, Poplar, Willow, etc.) may turn a fever into chills. Conversely, stimulating the fever, as with Elder or Yarrow, can prove excessive on occasion. Any reaction which itself denigrates or impedes the body's strength must be avoided, since one of the main validities of proper herb therapy is to aid and augment defense responses without hindering them with toxicities. Since the pharmacology of most herbs is so diffused, they are rarely focused enough to supplant or sidestep body defenses in the manner of some drugs. Although these same drugs will usually have distinct secondary toxicities, they often serve valid semiheroic functions where an individual has failed to regain internal equilibrium. Excessive quantities of an herb sufficient to cause a toxic reaction simply compromise basic health without the synthetic defenses offered by some drugs.

For chronic illness, more complex combinations are usually more effective than single remedies, with small regular doses preferable to erratic large portions. The dose should be small enough that no overt symptoms are produced. To facilitate the effectiveness of long-term maintenance remedies in chronic disease, a simple formula may be used. As an example, a person has a chronic pulmonary weakness, with a history of asthma as a child and a tendancy to have most common viral infections settle in the bronchials. This formula would go as follows:

1. SPECIFIC: (Yerba Santa, Grindelia, Inmortal, or Pleurisy Root)
2. LAXATIVE: (psyllium seed, Dandelion Root, etc.)
3. LIVER STIMULANT: (Burdock, Yellow Dock, Toadflax, etc.)
4. DIURETIC: (corn silk, Cleavers, etc.)
5. LYMPHATIC: (Red Root, echinacea, etc.)
6. NERVINE: (Skullcap, passion flower, etc.)

In conclusion, #1 should be an herb or herbs dealing with the chronic problem and should be the largest component. The rest, #s 2–6, are "satellite" herbs to facilitate and diffuse. None of the nonspecific herbs should be present in palpable

16

quantitites, that is, the laxative should not have a pronounced laxative effect, the nervine should not be strong enough to cause any drowsiness, and so forth. The rest of the formula is only to aid in making changes that can occur as a result of the specific. Unlike acute disease, the course of chronic illness is slow and usually submerged; therefore, treatment will always take weeks or months.

Further, most chronic problems not of direct genetic cause will generally derive from imbalances in life style, diet, emotional or spiritual instability, and stress. The end result (chronic disease) can be considered as a negative habit of body function or response. The best time to instigate therapy on any or all these levels, including herbal, is during periods of change. For some the spring or fall season is most auspicious, for others it can be moving to another place, leaving a relationship, a new child, or changing jobs, religions, or diet.

The combining of drug and herb therapy can be useful, useless, or disaster prone, and is far too unpredictable to deal with in great detail. An herb such as Alfalfa, with virtually no systemic effect other than as a source of soluble nutrients, is a useful adjunct to drug therapies, but otherwise it is safest to leave each to its separate realm. Some specific horrors should be mentioned, however. Like aspirin, the salicylate herbs should never be combined with anticoagulant drugs. These include Birch, Poplar, Willow, and probably even members of the Ericaceae order such as Blueberry, Pipsissewa, Pyrola, Manzanita, and Uva Ursi. Herbs with pronounced sedative effects, like their drug counterparts, should not be consumed with alcohol . . . or their drug counterparts. More complex and unpredictable drug approaches such as anticholinergics, adrenergic blocking agents, and the like should be taken under the closest supervision and not combined with any herb, since one can create a witches' brew of side effects. Herbs containing coumarin may be safe as teas (Sweet Clover, woodruff, etc.) but can become frankensteinian combinations with some drugs. A plant high in tannins will prevent or slow down absorption of drug substances or even precipitate them out completely. At the same time, laxative herbs or those effecting liver function may seriously alter the predictability of a drug action. Much study has gone into the fate and absorption rates of drug therapy, and doses are set based on normal metabolizations, with herbal laxatives and liver stimulants only interfering.

The time of day and mode of use affects the strength of reaction to many herbs. Sedatives and laxatives work best when their use coincides with normal patterns of sleep and defecation. A bitter tonic or stomachic works best when taken shortly before meals or predictable discomfort. Potential irritants, such as Bayberry or cayenne, should be taken on a full stomach, herbs meant to work quickly, on an empty stomach. An herb taken for recurring symptoms that give advance warning (such as migraine headaches) or are part of a predictable stress (such as insomnia or hangovers) works better when taken *before* the discomfort has ripened.

In dealing with young children a great deal of caution must be used, since body defences can quickly prove inadequate, and the speed at which an ailment can become dangerous is often foreshortened. In young children and infants, the speed of infection may not be quantitatively different than in an adult, but an organ or tissues can be compromised much sooner because of the considerably smaller volume of resistant tissue. One should be especially cautious in totally relying on home remedies for small children when the sickness is febrile (feverish), eruptive, or involves diarrhea or the eyes, ears, or mouth. Also, any lung infections should be approached conservatively. The most fanatically devout follower of natural healing methods should still take an infant or young child to a physician when there is any doubt at all, since the course of such diseases can be quick, volatile, and unpredictable. On the other hand, children respond very well to the simplest, most benign herb remedies. Seldom is anything stronger than Vervain necessary to bring them both palliative and substantive relief. Doses, of course, should be a half or a third as much.

Similarly, certain modifications should be used in treating the aged. They are usually more sensitive to herbs and drugs, and smaller quantities should be used, from one-half to two-thirds as much. Special care must be taken when an herb has a nauseating or cathartic effect. A safe quantity of Lobelia under other circumstances can induce a depressing, clammy nausea in an aged person; an energetic laxative may produce painful cramps and irritate the colon or small intestine. The equilibrium of health is often more delicate in the aged, with only small changes causing great discomfort. Most illness of age is the direct result of chronic disease, and herbal medications should be given using the formula under chronic disease therapy above.

Rare diseases *are* rare, and most discomforts and illnesses can be helped with herbs. Still, the ideal circumstance is to know (or be) a physician that will allow for the validity of herbal medicine yet act as a screen for more serious problems. Lacking that, get to know your body and use common sense. Even though a drug therapy may not always be the best approach, the best diagnostician for the nuts-and-bolts mechanistic problems of the body is a physician, the best judge for drug therapies is a pharmacist.

CULTIVATION: Wild plants are tricky. If you are serious, get a soil-testing kit, test for PH and such when getting wild plants, and duplicate those conditions in your garden. Land-grant universities in all states will analyze soil for only a modest fee. Further, if a plant likes slopes, prefers open meadows, or cloisters under bushes, duplicate that in your garden. Learn to observe the growing conditions of the healthy plants in the wild. If you are going to transplant roots, get them after all the above-ground plant has died back, and get *all* the root. If the plant grows in the high mountains and you are gathering mature seeds, pack them in native soil, put them in your freezer, and alternate freezing with defrosting several times until the seeds start to germinate. In some plants this can take a year or more, while others will start to sprout in your freezer. Yet other plants will simply rot no matter what you do. As a rule of thumb, common plants are easiest to cultivate; uncommon ones are probably scarce because of their adaptation to very specific and narrow conditions. Members of the orchid family are always a lost cause, and those of the lily family may demand heroic efforts, so good luck.

18

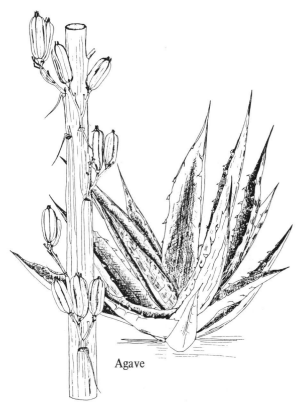

Agave

AGAVE

Agave spp.   Liliaceae

OTHER NAMES: Century Plant, Maguey

APPEARANCE: Similar to Yucca and often mistaken for it, Agave is a more robust plant with broader, thicker spiney-edged leaves and a flowering stalk that, unlike Yucca, forms armlike branches.

HABITAT: From 2,000 to 7,000 feet on mesa sides, limestone slopes, and rocky mountainsides; throughout the West in higher desert and rough terrain.

COLLECTING: Leaves, Method A; deep taproots, Method B.

MEDICINAL USE: The leaves and particularly the root contain the sapogenins hecogenin and tigogenin, soapy substances used in manufacturing steroids. A teaspoon of the expressed leaf sap or one-fourth ounce of the dried leaf boiled in tea helps indigestion, stomach fermentation, and chronic constipation. The fresh sap is used for burns, cuts, and skin abrasions. The root, fresh or dried, makes a useful soap and, like Yucca, has been used for arthritis — one-half teaspoon of the root powder in tea, morning and evening. Constant use may interfere with oil-soluble vitamin absorption in the small intestine. In Mexico it has also been used for jaundice, in similar doses.

19

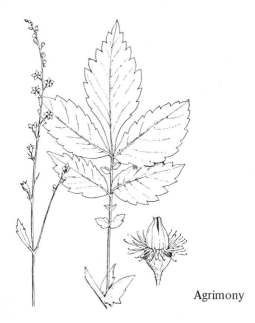

Agrimony

AGRIMONY

Agrimonia gryposepala Rosaceae

APPEARANCE: A member of the rose family, with foot-long thin terminal racemes of numerous yellow flowers, five petaled and roselike, maturing into little round burrs. The basal leaves are shaped like mustard greens; hairy and pinnate, with the three terminal leaflets the largest, the inner ones of varying sizes. The two- to three-foot stem has smaller, irregular leaves, usually three parted.

HABITAT: Middle mountains of southern California, particularly the San Bernardino, Palomar, and San Jacinto ranges and the north central sections of Arizona, in Yellow Pine or Ponderosa forests.

COLLECTING: The whole plant, bundled, Method A.

MEDICINAL USE: An astringent and diuretic, containing mallic acid and tannin, with some oxalic acid in the root. A teaspoon of the dried root or tablespoon of the herb is drunk as needed for urine acidity and mild bladder and urethra inflammations. Internally and externally for mild hives and moist skin eruptions. A weak tea of the leaves is a soothing eyewash. Once used for jaundice, probably because of the yellow flowers, and a yellow dye once made from the root.

ALFALFA

Medicago sativa Leguminosae

OTHER NAMES: Lucerne

APPEARANCE: For all appearances a tall clover, with three-part leaves. The plant is a many stemmed and branched perennial, usually two to three feet tall when mature. The flowers are like typical clovers, with purple, lavender, or blue tufts of blossoms interspersed at the ends of the stems. It is very difficult to differentiate

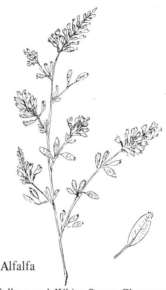

Alfalfa

between Alfalfa and Yellow and White Sweet Clover until they are in bloom, although Yellow Sweet Clover grows earlier and White Sweet Clover is larger. It is a ridiculously common plant in cultivation in the United States both for crop rotation and fodder, but most people have never seen an Alfalfa plant in bloom . . . it's rather pretty.

HABITAT: Feral plants in the West are found most commonly in foothills and mountains (3,000–9,000 feet), where they prefer moist soil in dry areas and drier soil in moist areas. Abundant when located, but not widely dispersed.

COLLECTING: The whole upper half of the plant (Method A) when just blooming, if possible a week or two after rain. The leaves and flowers are the only parts used and, as densely stemmed as Alfalfa is, a combination of stripping and shaking is the best cleaning method. The little sharp leaves (stipules) at the base of the leaf stem are rather sharp and can scratch the skin unless reasonable care (or a glove) is used.

MEDICINAL USE: Not really medicinal at all (although a cup of hot tea when you feel bad certainly does *some* good), Alfalfa tea should be classed more as a food, or at least a dietary aid. Alfalfa chooses fairly rich soil where it grows by choice and is an indicator of dirt that is relatively high in minerals. Much commercially available Alfalfa tea is a by-product of farming and is raised in a fairly cruddy environment. Alfalfa tea is hardly a taste sensation when purchased from stores, at best resembling the taste of sun-dried grass clippings, at worst a coloring agent for hot water. Wild Alfalfa actually *has* a taste. It still mixes best with a little mint or lemon grass. The high mineral content of the tea, particularly calcium and trace minerals, along with Vitamin K and Folic Acid, make it an excellent recuperative aid, as well as a small but appreciable adjunct to the diet for chronic and functional illnesses such as arthritis and rheumatism, colitis, ulcers, anemia, etc. It is a traditional European and Russian tea for wasting diseases and is used in some German clinics as a dietary aid in Celiac Disease, together with traditional treatment and diet. A safe and appropriate tea for pregnancy, along with Raspberry leaves; also good to drink when sulfa or antibiotic drugs are taken.

ALUM ROOT

Heuchera spp.   Saxifragaceae

OTHER NAMES: Mountain Saxifrage

APPEARANCE: This is a pretty little plant, easily overlooked unless in flower. The root is large, scaly from dead growth, and usually angled out or even downward from rock crevices; it is dark barked and the inner pith is flesh colored or pink, with an intensely astringent taste. The leaves are basal in all of our species, ranging from one-half to two inches across. They are shallow lobed and round, resembling those of garden geraniums, with the stem indented into the base of the leaf. The many small flowers, blooming intermittently throughout the summer, are borne on leafless spikes, from one to six from a single root. They will often cluster along one side of the stem, and range from pinkish white to light green. *H. sanguinea* of southern Arizona has crimson flowers. Flowering is of short duration, and most of the time all that is visible are the clusters of basal leaves.

HABITAT: In the West, Alum Root is a high mountain plant, needing much moisture, shade, and rich mulch. It is most frequently encountered in wet rocks and down moist embankments and slopes, generally on a north or south side. The various species are usually in abundance in the upper reaches of our highest mountains, often growing up to, and beyond, timberline. In southern California, Alum Root is found in the highest peaks of the San Bernardino and San Gabriel ranges as well as the Sierra Nevadas. In Arizona, Nevada, Colorado, and New Mexico it grows at higher elevations, in mountains that exceed 9,000 feet, although sometimes encountered much lower. In Wyoming and Montana, plants may descend to 5,000 feet.

COLLECTING: The roots should be cut from the green part of the plant, washed, and the dead scales removed with a stiff brush. Use Method B.

MEDICINAL USE: Alum Root is one of our strongest astringents, containing up to twenty percent tannin. Its overall effect, however, is less irritating than Cranesbill, Oak Bark, or Cañaigre. A teaspoon of the chopped root, boiled in water for twenty minutes, can be used for gastroenteritis ("stomach flu"), particularly with symptoms of diarrhea and dry, bilious vomiting. The tea makes an excellent gargle for sore throats, especially when combined with one-fourth teaspoon of golden seal root; a half cup drunk an hour before every meal will stimulate the healing of regenerating ulcers of the esophagus and stomach, but of little use for duodenal ulcers. The root is an old folk remedy for dysentery, a cup drunk every two hours for at least a day. Since most astringents (tannin, malic acid, catechol, etc.) are precipitated before reaching the colon, obstinate dysentery should be treated by an enema; a teaspoon of the chopped root boiled for twenty minutes in a pint of water. The same quantity can be used as a douche for vaginitis or mild cervicitis (Pap Class I or II, without dysplasia). The finely ground root is a good first aid for treating cuts and abrasions, promoting almost instant clotting; if combined with equal parts golden seal root and *Echinacea angustifolia* root, the mixture makes an excellent antiseptic powder.

CULTIVATION: The plant requires a very moist but well drained area in a garden or greenhouse, with at least seventy percent shade. Cultivated from root division in spring or fall, and does best when surrounded by some mulch from the original area.

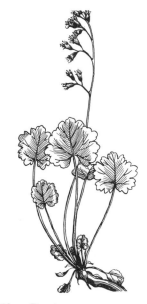

Alum Root

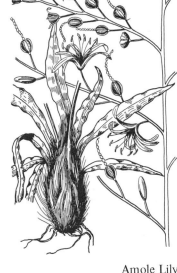

Amole Lily

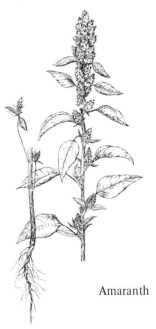

Amaranth

AMARANTH

Amaranthus spp.   Amaranthaceae

OTHER NAMES: Red Cockscomb, Alegria, Love-Lies-Bleeding, Pigweed

APPEARANCE: The more noticeable features of the Amaranths, including many tropical escapees now found abundantly at all altitudes, are the many dense spikes of inconspicuous flowers, the immense numbers of little shiny dark seeds a plant can produce, and the common habit of the Amaranths to become reddish stemmed upon maturity. The leaves are alternate, oblong or long-stemmed oval, bright green and, in upright species, from one to three inches long. The plants are highly adaptable, growing three inches high with one little tuft of flowers or six feet and still growing, if supplied with good soil, moisture, and sun. The upright Amaranths are the more useful medicinally, and the redder the stem the stronger the effects. Cultivated Amaranths (Red Cockscomb, for one) have striking blood red or maroon flowers and stems, but most wild escapees are much more subdued. If it is one or two feet high, growing along roads or disturbed earth, has no bright or obvious flower, and generally resembles the penultimate weed, it's either a *Chenopodium* (goosefoot) or an Amaranth (pigweed). Some species of Amaranth have reddish dots or lighter spots in the middle of the leaves.

HABITAT: Almost anywhere, although those of our mountains, with shorter growing seasons and a more defined climate, are more useful medicinally.

COLLECTING: In full bloom or seed, Method A. Plants that still retain full green leaves but with pronounced reddening of the stems are preferable. If the little seeds are to be harvested for grain, the bundles should be hung over newspaper while drying, and the spikes shaken periodically to loosen the seeds. More complete gleaning can be accomplished by throwing the dried spikes into a blender and winnowing in a deep bowl or through a strainer. Young green plants are an excellent pot herb.

MEDICINAL USES: The main function of Amaranth is as a pleasant, mild astringent for the mucus membranes. A strong tea (tablespoon of chopped leaves in a cup) can be drunk every several hours for mild stomach and intestinal irritation, particularly the recuperative period of gastroenteritis or stomach flu to lessen irritability of the tissues. It will aid in mild diarrhea and hemorrhoid and pile inflammation. A douche made with a handful of the leaves in a pint of water will aid vaginal itching and inflammation without accompanying discharge. A few dried leaves and a teaspoon of lavender flowers or chamomile flowers steeped for ten minutes in hot milk and cooled can be given to an infant with colic or ejectile vomiting. The fresh plant has little medicinal value, other than using for a cooling poultice. Only the dried plant has an appreciable amount of astringency.

OTHER USES: Several varieties of Amaranth have shown major promise as a crop plant. The little seeds are nourishing and the strains grow well in otherwise useless crop lands, adapted to alkaline, low-nitrogen soils.

CULTIVATION: Red Cockscomb, an old favorite of gardeners, should be purchased from nursery stock or grown from commercial seed. The fecund wild varieties are to be avoided like the plague; fertile, scruffy, and adaptable to any soil, from cow pastures to dirty thumbnails.

AMOLE LILY

Chlorogalum spp.   Liliaceae

OTHER NAMES: Soap Plant, Soap Lily

APPEARANCE: A small California lily, with a basal rosette of long, thin wavy leaves and a single one-to two-foot stem formed in early summer. It is leafless, with several white or pink, widely spaced blossoms. The bulb is covered with a dense coat of brown hair, the inner pith soapy and cream colored and with a mild onionlike scent.

HABITAT: Rocky hillsides throughout California, especially the southern half, from 1,500 to 5,500 feet and even lower in the ocean-facing coastal ranges. Usually found in stands of well spaced plants.

COLLECTING: The hairy bulbs at any time, used fresh or allowed to dry, which can take months. Usually difficult to identify until summer, when annual grasses have died back, exposing the long basal leaves. By mid autumn, however, the leaves have died back.

MEDICINAL USE: Contains the saponin chlorogenin, which kills or stuns fish but leaves the flesh edible. Amole Lily makes a shampoo or skin soap useful for cradle cap, smelly dandruff, or skin rashes under beards or eyebrows. Use as the only soap for these areas until the condition clears up, grating the husked bulb into one-half cup hot water until there is enough to form a suds.

CULTIVATION: The live bulb can be planted in a similar environment at any time but seeds poorly in cultivation.

ANGELICA

Angelica spp.   Umbelliferae

OTHER NAMES: Archangel, Oshá del Campo

APPEARANCE: Angelica is a stout, hollow-stemmed plant, from two to four or five feet high, with a passing resemblance to its more delicate relative, celery. The large leaves are divided into smaller ones, usually about two inches long, either smooth or finely hairy on the underside, and oval to cutleaf in shape. The whole plant has a strong, peculiar odor, typically Angelica, which resembles a cross between celery and Juniper and is strongest in the root and seeds. Lower parts of the plant may have a slight purplish tinge, particularly in the autumn, but should not be confused with poison hemlock, a much more delicate plant with carrotlike leaves and purple or wine-colored splotches on the base of the stems. The flowers form the usual inverted umbrellalike umbel characteristic of the family. They are white, maturing into double seeds which, when separated, are egg shaped, completely flat on the inner side, and strongly ridged and convex on the outer. The large, fleshy root is medium brown with a cream-colored pith and strong, slightly soapy smell.

HABITAT: Although not a common plant in our area, it is widespread in higher elevations. Not a people plant, it frequents rather inaccessible areas. *A. tomentosa* is sporadic in the coastal mountains of California from San Diego north, and, unlike other species, may grow as low as 1,500 feet and as high as 6,000 feet in moist, shady places. Other species are found at higher elevations, almost to timberline, in the Sierra Nevadas and in Arizona south of the Mogollon Escarpment, the Kaibab Plateau, and Lukachukai area, as well as the higher elevations of Nevada and Utah. In New Mexico (*A. pinnata*) and southern Colorado (*A. pinnata* and *A. grayi*) Angelica can range from dry high valleys to slopes on the western side of the

Rockies to the rain forests between 10,000 feet and timberline. *A. hendersonii* is a common plant of coastal bluffs from central California, northwards.

COLLECTING: Angelica is a big plant and many large stands can be found in our area, but, because of its reclusive habits, it is probably wise to check with an herbarium for locations. I have spent days hiking (and gasping) after Angelica in some probable location, only to find, two years later, a stand of hundreds of ancient plants around the next mountainside. The large roots should be washed, split, and dried (Method B), the leaves bundled by the long stems (Method A), and the seeds dried on the stems (Method C) to be rubbed off before storing.

MEDICINAL USES: Angelica serves a number of functions. In regulating poor digestion the root and seeds are used frequently, in small quantities — a scant teaspoon in a cup of water. This should be *boiled* for an aromatic bitter and *steeped* for an anesthetic and astringent to the stomach lining. A tincture of the root or seeds acts as an antispasmodic for intestinal cramps ranging from simple nausea to tenesmus. To prevent cramping from cathartic herbs or medicines, one-fourth teaspoon is drunk in warm water. Because of a complex pharmacology, ranging from volatile and fixed oils to phytosterols and saponins, Angelica has a varying solubility in water, and can have different effects when taken as a boiled tea, steeped tea, tincture, or capsule. The seeds in a tincture should be kept in the medicine chest as a first aid for nausea, stomach cramps, and intestinal irritability (one-half teaspoon in four ounces warm water) or in small, frequent doses for bladder or urethra inflammations (one-fourth teaspoon in eight ounces warm water). A tea of the chopped root is useful as a sedative in feverish irritability and for any "hot" illness. It also acts as a menstrual stimulant and antispasmodic for cramps, whether the bleeding is heavy or light . . . in effect, helping to regulate menstruation. The well-known Chinese herbal remedy, dong-kwai or tang-kuei (so-called "woman's ginseng"), is a cured and processed root derived from several species, and is used as a general female tonic, although equally useful for such male problems as prostatitis and orchitis. The roots or seeds in tea, tincture, or capsule have an effect very similar to that of Oshá, stimulating both sweat and sebaceous secretions in fevers, cooling the skin and generally stimulating defense mechanisms at the onset of a viral infection.

OTHER USES: The dried leaves have a pleasant parsleylike scent and serve as a vegetable or fish spice and a good salad garnish. They are used in the making of Vermouth and Chartreuse. The candied stalks of European Angelica are a confectioner's standby. The American species can be treated similarly, but traditional English and French preserving methods are so tortuous that, to save space, the avid candied Angelica fancier is referred hereby to *A Modern Herbal*, Volume I, by Grieve, where several Byzantine recipes are included for this peculiar substance.

CULTIVATION: The roots should be dusted with a hormone, divided, and planted at any time, the freshly dried seeds sown the same fall, with the thinnest of cover. Angelica likes rich, moist but well-drained soil.

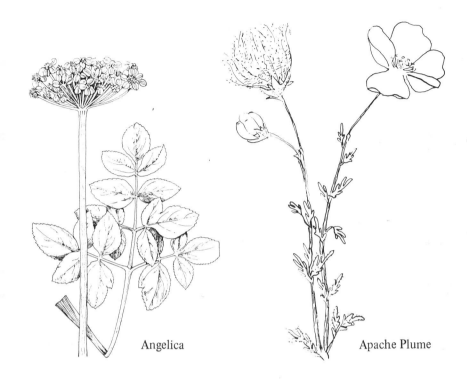

Angelica   Apache Plume

APACHE PLUME

Fallugia paradoxa   Rosaceae

OTHER NAMES: Poñil

APPEARANCE: A medium-sized, thinly branched bush, the stems whitish silvery in new growth, shreddy in older. The tiny silvery green leaves are palmate to pinnate; the flowers are snow white and roselike, maturing into flesh-colored plumes of seeds that fancifully resemble the plume on an Apache war bonnet . . . whatever that is. Plumes intermingle with new flowers throughout the growing season—the "paradox" of the Latin name. Unlike many similar waist-high gray green sagebrush, Apache Plume is deciduous, dropping its leaves in late autumn, regenerating in spring.

HABITAT: Juniper/Piñon belts from the eastern borders of the higher Mohave Desert, through Nevada and all points eastward to the Texas hill country, from 4,000 to 7,500 feet.

MEDICINAL USE: According to Curtin, the roots dug in the fall are boiled in water for coughs, drunk morning and evening, and the tea used as a hair rinse after shampooing. The powdered root (with tobacco) or the flowers (with Horehound and flour) are used for painful joints or soft tissue swellings, applied locally as a poultice or fomentation. The spring twigs may be boiled and drunk for indigestion and "spring" fevers.

27

ARNICA

Arnica spp.   Compositeae

OTHER NAMES: Leopardsbane

APPEARANCE: These are sunflowerlike flowers, bright yellow, with foliage that is usually strongly scented and opposite leaves that may be alternate directly below the flowers, their shapes varying from lance-to heart-shaped. Generally not much taller than two feet, but otherwise a fairly substantial plant with large flowers, leaves, and roots.

HABITAT: High mountains, from timberline down to 9,000 feet, somewhat lower in the San Bernardino ranges in California. One of what botanists refer to as DYCs (Damn Yellow Compositeaes), an expression of benign disgust from a master and of abject terror from a student, since it seems that (subjectively) fully two-thirds of all plants form yellow blossoms resembling a cross between Dandelion and sunflower. It is said that only elder, revered Masters, with manes of snow white hair and countenances of beatific confusion, are privy to their divers names, and many a Bedlam is filled with students mumbling hoarsely *"Acamptopappus, Aplopappus, Achyrachaena, Agoseris, Amblyopappus,"* a sad litany of DYCs. Although in some areas Arnicas may descend to lower altitudes, into a confusion of similar appearing plants, in the relative tranquility of subalpine and alpine zones they are more easily recognized, and more common.

MEDICINAL USE: Arnica is an external remedy, with the fresh (or wilted) plant used, root and all. An amount of rubbing alcohol, equal to three times the volume of chopped plant, is steeped for a week and squeezed through a cloth. This liniment can be used freely for joint inflammations, sprains, and sore muscles. If the tincture causes a slight skin irritation, dilute with an equal quantity of rubbing alcohol. The strengths of the various unofficial Arnicas are variable in terms of volatile oils, sterols, and glycosides and should not be strong enough to cause excessive reddening of normal skin. A hot rag dipped in the liniment can be used as a counterirritant . Arnica as a tea is too strong for safe internal use and can cause blistering of the intestinal mucosa.

ASPARAGUS

Asparagus officinale   Liliaceae (Asparagaceae)

APPEARANCE AND HABITAT: This is the Asparagus of commerce, found wild in all areas of the Rocky Mountains, in higher elevations of northern Arizona, Utah, and Nevada (from 5,500 feet to 8,000 feet), and usually in rural or farming areas. The spring shoots are the familiar Asparagus stalks. Asparagus Ferns are generally somewhat more decorative and petite varieties of the above, used similarly, at least if you want to cannibalize your houseplant. They can be found once in awhile growing wild in the older sections of Los Angeles, Santa Barbara, and such places, along embankments and moist inner city hillsides. The official species does appear infrequently near Ojai and Ventura. It is a toughly branched, small stemmed plant of three or four feet, usually with several branches sprouting from the same rootstalk, the branches often in various stages of growth. Its only leaves are degenerate scales at the joints of the stems. The flowers are little solitary bells, snow white, maturing into currant-sized red berries containing shiny black seeds. The roots are long and many branched, sometimes attaining considerable size. Even a small, coherent piece of root will regrow the next year if left in the ground.

28

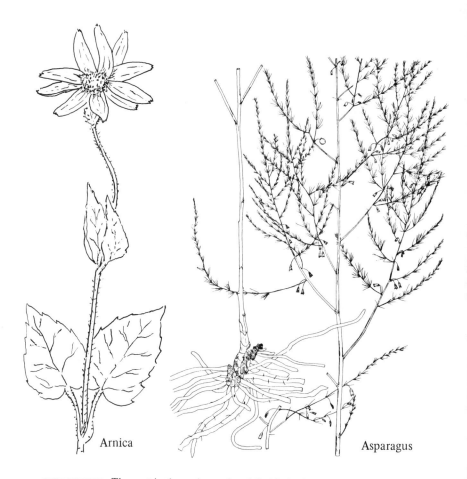

Arnica

Asparagus

COLLECTING: The root in the spring or late fall, Method B or C, depending on the root size.

MEDICINAL USE: A diuretic and laxative. The peculiar smell of post-Asparagus urine is from the sulphur compound methanethiol (methyl mercaptan), also found in radishes. The diuretic effect is strong and persistent, with no ill effect on healthy kidneys but having the likelihood of aggravating kidney inflammation. A tea, made from one to two teaspoons of the chopped root, is useful for gout and urate-related joint inflammations and helps prevent related kidney stones. May be useful in general for acquired hyperuricemia, but probably of little value when the condition is hereditary. The same tea is also a gentle but effective laxative where an irritating cathartic would be inappropriate, such as with the bedridden, elderly, or pregnant. In pregnancy, the kidney stimulation could be undesirable during the last trimester for some women.

AVENS

Geum spp.   Rosaceae

APPEARANCE: The flowers are few, roselike, and terminal, generally yellow or flesh colored. The calyx teeth are five, like the petals, and sometimes purplish, becoming plumed or burrlike when in seed. The leaves are long, pinnate, and lyrelike, with the terminal lobes large, the middle lobes smaller and sometimes almost reduced to tufted scales, the leaves on the flowering stems simpler, usually three or five parted. Easily confused with Agrimony, the latter having a similar two or three foot height and also hairy, but possessing long terminal spikes of many small flowers, in contrast to a maximum of six or eight for Avens. The leaves of Avens are also longer, with more reduced mid-leaflets, and the plant overall, except for the fruit, has a somewhat Raspberrylike visage.

HABITAT: Throughout our range, generally in pleasant, middle-altitude forest meadows, amidst and above the Ponderosa belt, usually near water.

COLLECTING: The herb, Method A; the root, Method B.

MEDICINAL USE: One of our better dysentery remedies. A tablespoon of the chopped root, boiled in a cup of milk or water and sipped on for several hours, with two or three cups a day usually necessary. In treating a pink and smelly vaginal discharge, a tablespoon of the root in tea drunk during the course of the day for several days will generally stop the flow. For uterine hemorrhage, excessive menstruation, and middle-of-the-month spotting, two tablespoons of the root boiled in a quart of water for twenty minutes and drunk in small doses during a day is generally effective, and may be continued for two or three days if necessary. If a substantial flare-up of the bleeding occurs the day after stopping the tea, or if it does not subside in a rational length of time, a pelvic examination is probably in order. Avens is also a good tea for inflammation and irritability of the stomach lining—a rounded teaspoon of the herb or a scant teaspoon of the root is drunk between meals.

BANEBERRY   (see color plate)

Actaea arguta   Ranunculaceae

APPEARANCE: This is a large perennial herb, with big erect basal leaves divided in threes, interspersed with flowering stalks, all arising from a dark brown rootstalk. The flowers form cream-colored, delicate oval puffs in the early summer, maturing to terminal masses of red berries that form an oval cluster. Some plants form white pearllike berries, a genetic anomaly, but are otherwise identical.

HABITAT: Moist, rich woods, usually in shade. Higher altitudes of the San Bernardino ranges and the Sierra Nevada, through Arizona and New Mexico northwards, generally above or in the upper reaches of the Ponderosa belt. Common.

COLLECTING: The roots, Method B, ground when dry.

MEDICINAL USE: It is an acrid irritant and moderately poisonous internally, depressing vagus function, with cardiac arrest possible from large doses. The powdered root is a good counterirritant, the powder mixed with hot water, applied where appropriate , and covered with hot towels. If used with an excess of verve, blistering is possible.

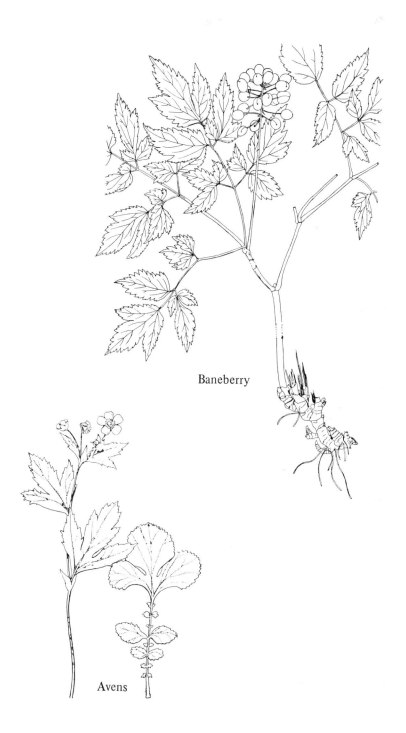

Baneberry

Avens

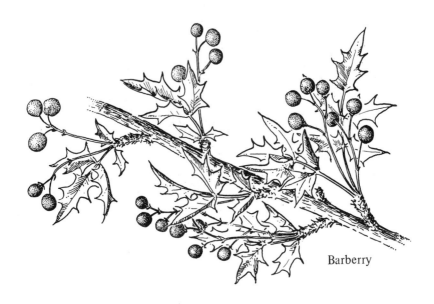

Barberry

BARBERRY

Mahonia (Berberis) fremontii, B. fendleri   Berberidaceae

OTHER NAMES: Hollygrape, Palo Amarillo, Mahonia

APPEARANCE: All Barberry plants are spiny . . . somewhere. The most common species throughout our area is Fremont's or Desert Barberry, a stout shrub with yellow wood and spiny, hollylike leaves that are arranged in fives or sevens. Flowers are in little grapelike bright yellow bunches, blooming in late spring and early summer, ripening into somewhat inflated berries, dull purple in higher elevations, dull brown in the desert, with a taste both slightly sweet and intensely bitter. Stems are from three to ten feet tall, and the plants usually form irregular clusters or small stands. The single most distinctive aspect of any Barberry is the bright, almost fluorescent yellow rootwood. No exception, the other more common Barberry is *Berberis fendleri,* a plant closely resembling the Common Barberry of Europe (which itself is found wild on occasion). The leaves are smooth and oblong-oval, occurring in little clusters along the stem, each cluster accompanied by three needle-thin spikes. The flowers are also bright yellow, turning to little scarlet currant-sized berries that droop from one side of the two- to four-foot stems. Other species have berries from light yellow to blue.

HABITAT: *Berberis fendleri* is a plant of the Rockies, usually from 6,000 to 9,000 feet, a plant of coniferous hillsides. Fremont's Barberry is found in drier canyons and foothills, usually below the Juniper/Piñon belts in New Mexico and Arizona, down into the dry foothills of the Colorado and Mohave deserts of California. A Texas species, Algerita, with only three spiny leaflets, is found in the foothills of southern Arizona and New Mexico as well. There are several other bush Barberries of a similar appearance in the California coastal ranges and the west slopes of the Sierra Nevadas.

32

COLLECTING: The roots at anytime, although best in late fall, dried loosely in a paper box or bag. The flowers or berries when still alive, Method C.

MEDICINAL USE: The physiological effects of Barberry are primarily due to the presence of the yellow alkaloid berberine, the intensely bitter coloring agent of the root. It follows that the stronger the color of the root, the more potent it is. Barberry is one of the most beneficial medicinal plants of the West, useful as an antipyretic for lowering fevers and inflammatory conditions, as a laxative and intestinal strengthener, as an antibacterial skin wash, and as a liver stimulant and "blood purifier." For fevers, mucosa inflammations, and stomach bitter and intestinal "tonic," one-half teaspoon boiled in eight ounces of water for ten minutes can be drunk every three to four hours, or a tablespoon can be boiled in a quart of water for a day's supply, sipped periodically. A slightly rounded teaspoon of the root drunk in the evening generally will have a laxative effect by morning, acting as a stimulant to peristalsis. The same dose can be an excellent hangover treatment the morning after. For individuals with a history of hepatitis and who suffer occasional bilirubin elevations, a tablespoon of Barberry and a tablespoon of Toadflax boiled together in a quart of water and drunk during the day for several days can generally return the blood to normal. The flowers make an excellent skin dressing to prevent infection, and a teaspoon of the berries in tea can be used for fevers, as a laxative, and for gum inflammations.

OTHER USES: The fruit of some Barberry species is sweet and sour enough to make a pleasant preserve. Most are too bitter, however.

CULTIVATION: Several varieties are available from nurseries. If wild stock is desired, dig when dormant in the fall, pack in wet sand, and plant six inches deep in the late fall.

BAYBERRY

Myrica californica   Myricaceae

OTHER NAMES: Wax Myrtle, California Sweet Bay

APPEARANCE AND HABITAT: This shrub or small tree is found all along the lower western ridges of the California coastal ranges, from the Santa Monica Mountains north to British Columbia, sometimes descending nearly to the surf. The plant is sometimes confused with California Bay, a true tree of larger dimensions and broader, more widely spaced leaves emitting an overwhelmingly strong scent when crushed. Bayberry has many shiny, dark green leaves, oval-lanceolate, with a slight, pleasant spicy scent. The fruit are brownish purple, waxy coated and about one-third of an inch in diameter, growing in clusters along the slender branches. The thin bark is a grayish brown.

COLLECTING: The root bark is the major part (although the tree bark is serviceable), and this is collected in late fall. In many areas only solitary small trees are encountered sporadically, and the temptation to take a few large surface roots should be resisted; they don't usually survive such compromise harvesting, as I have found out. Wait until a stand is found and dig up a complete individual. The whole root mass is removed, washed, and the larger roots pounded until the bark separates, the smaller rootlets used in their entirety. The leaves make a pleasant tea when brewed lightly, and slightly expectorant. As to the seeds, they may be used like Juniper berries for flavouring strong meat, but most particularly are a source for a good ointment or candle wax. As much as one and one-half pounds of wax can be harvested from a tree-bush. The berries are crushed and dropped into boiling water; the melting point of the wax is from 120 to 130 degrees farenheit. When a batch of berries has been exhausted of wax, ice cubes can be thrown in the water or the whole pot allowed to cool until the wax hardens enough to lift out. It makes yellowish or green smokeless aromatic candles as well as a fine-lathering astringent soap.

MEDICINAL USES: The root bark (and the tree bark, for that matter) is an effective vasodilator for the skin and intestinal mucosa, and often used in conjunction with capsicum to stimulate a more rapid healing of mucosa infections or inflammations by increasing the circulation of blood and lymph and helping to prevent the inefficient poorly drained engorgements of sinus and stomach membranes many people are prone to. A capsule of capsicum and a scant teaspoon of Bayberry can be surprisingly effective in warding off a cold if taken at the first feeble signs of onset. A tablespoon of the bark in a pint of water, drunk regularly in small amounts during the day, will promote healing of stomach and small and large intestine irritations and ulcerations, speeding the tissue healing and preventing overinflammatory conditions. Although not usually as effective as the official species of present herbal use and former drug use *(M. cerifera* of the eastern states), the latter, as it is usually found in commerce, is often a flaccid, expensive, and improperly handled crude drug of indeterminate age and potency. Many of the more important botanicals not presently used in drug manufacturing, particularly those from the eastern states, have not sustained a demand until the last five or ten years sufficient to keep many experienced pickers in the industry, with a resultant decrease in quality in many traditional botanical drugs. This being the case, the individual picking California Bayberry will end up with a better remedy than is available from a health food store or herb store. Although somewhat inelegant, swallowing a small piece of the berry wax (about the size of a lima bean) or chewing a few dried berries will exert an astringent and narcotic effect useful in treating dysentery and colitis, as well as dry, frantic coughs in older children.

BETONY (see color plate)

Pedicularis spp.   Scrophulariaceae

OTHER NAMES: Lousewort, Indian Warrior, Elephant Head, "Wood Betony"

APPEARANCE AND HABITAT: Betony is a member of the Figwort family, and bears a certain resemblance to its better known relatives the snapdragons. The overall form of the leaves is oval-lanceolate, with the margins ranging from only finely serrated to feathery and fernlike. The plants are usually found at the highest elevations of major ranges in a moist, rain forest environment. A major exception is the Indian Warrior *(P. densiflora)* of California which is found in the San Bernardino and coastal ranges from Los Angeles County northward, frequenting open hillsides. With California Poppy and lupine it forms those virulent displays of color in late April and early May that California is so famous for. Most Betonies are found above 7,500 feet, however, and many are considered as partial root parasites of some conifers; they are encountered on slopes, hollows, wet gorges, and shaded hillsides, often directly under older firs, spruces, or pines. The flowers form terminal clusters on the several stems and are distinctly shaped, the lower petals fused into a three-lobed "apron," the upper petal arching down or up, often snoutlike. Those formerly classed in the separate genera "Chelone" differ by the upper petal's forming a curved hood over the reduced lower petals. There are four

34

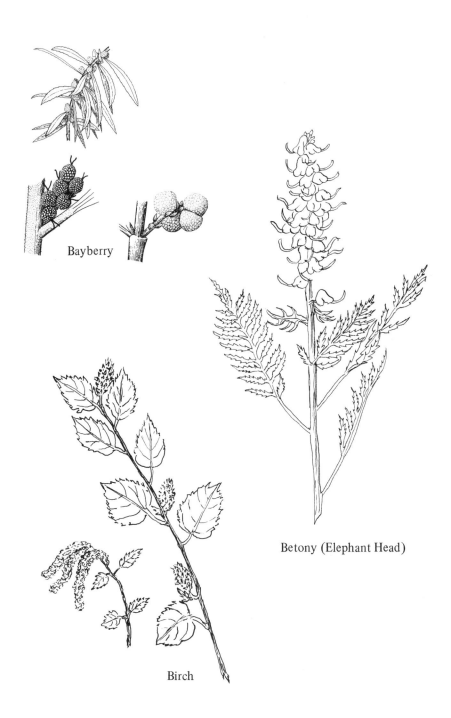

Bayberry

Betony (Elephant Head)

Birch

stamens. Both the flowers and foliage have only a slight odor, if any. Blossoms may be yellow green to cream or red to dark lavender purple. The big fernlike Elephant's Head *(P. groenlandica)* is one of the more spectacular plants of the high mountains, with its long, fernlike basal leaves, single two- or three-foot stem, and bright red elephantlike flowers, the single-fused upper petal sweeping down and forward like a tiny trunk between the lower petals which resemble ears. Betony, in general, frequents higher, moist mountains throughout the West, well above the Ponderosa belt.

COLLECTING: The whole flowering stalks, Method A or C, depending on stem length (often well under a foot) and the proportion of basal leaves.

MEDICINAL USES: *Pedicularis* is often confused, both in herb books and usage, with the Wood Betony *(Stachys betonica)* of Europe, an unrelated member of the mint family. Fortunately, their uses are very similar. Betony is an effective sedative for children and a tranquilizer for adults, particularly in hyperactive states (at all ages) that result from a generally frenzied day. It acts as a mild relaxant for skeletal muscles and the cerebrum, quieting anxieties and tension. The herb in tea, one-half to one teaspoon for children, a rounded teaspoon to tablespoon for adults. Betony also acts to stimulate sweating and will help reduce body temperature in fevers. The fresh or dried plant is a useful vulnerary for minor injuries, with mild astringent and antiseptic properties. Large quantities may cause a befuddled lethargy and some interference with motor control, particularly in the legs. It wouldn't hurt to test a particular collection before administering freely, since the potency of the various species is variable. In any respect, a moderate overdose causes only short term discomfort of minor consequence.

BIRCH

Betula fontinalis   Betulaceae

OTHER NAMES: Water Birch

APPEARANCE: This is a handsome small tree of watersides, with dark bronze, shiny bark, many slender branches, and resinous, knobby light-colored glands along the twigs. The leaves are oval and serrated, alternate, smooth but distinctly veined. The catkins may be an inch long, forming little winged nutlets. Birch can be confused with its relative white alder, the latter having light-colored bark, wavy leaves, smoother stems, and stiff, rounder pine-cone-like fruit.

HABITAT: Streamsides and moist places. In California it only reaches as far south as Inyo County in the southern Sierra Nevada, Panamint, and Inyo ranges, but common above 7,000 feet in Arizona and from the Manzano Mountains northwards in the Rockies.

COLLECTING: The leaves, Method A; the bark, Method D.

MEDICINAL USES: The leaves are a diuretic, best in small, frequent doses; the bark contains sufficient methyl salicylate to make it useful as a mild analgesic for headache and arthritis, as well as a hair rinse to stimulate growth. A tincture in rubbing alcohol of the bark makes an above average liniment.

BISTORT

Polygonum bistortoides   Polygonaceae

APPEARANCE AND HABITAT: This is a common plant of high alpine wet meadows, forming broad, widely dispersed stands above 10,000 feet. It has long, lance-shaped basal leaves and a few sheathing leaves of diminishing size along the one-to two-foot stalks. The flowers are little delicate terminal puffs of white to light pink flowers. The creeping horizontal roots are thick, fleshy, with a chaffy darker surface and small undersided thread roots.

COLLECTING: The whole roots, Method B (or C); ground after drying.

MEDICINAL USES: A strong astringent with antiseptic properties. The ground root, mixed with equal volumes of echinacea, golden seal, Oshá, or Yerba Mansa powdered roots, makes an excellent first aid dressing or antiseptic powder for cuts, scrapes, and the like. Mixed with clay or comfrey root it forms a good drawing poultice for abscesses, sprained joints, even injured tendons or broken fingers; enough hot water is added to form a mush and applied either open or under a hot cloth, changed every two or three hours. Can be used in teaspoon amounts in tea wherever internal astringency is needed. Bistort is especially useful for mouth lesions, bleeding gums, and patchy sore throats. The high-altitude packer that awakes in the morning with a distended or relaxed uvula (usually a mouth breather) will find that chewing on a fresh or dried Bistort root will shrink it and get rid of that half-swallowed slippery-choking sensation.

BLUEBERRY

Vaccinium spp.   Ericaceae

OTHER NAMES: Bilberry, Huckleberry, Whortleberry, California Blueberry, etc.

APPEARANCE AND HABITAT: The common names of this genera are varied and unreliable, with Huckleberries picked in thickets in Virginia but Blueberries (the same species) picked in Arkansas and the same plant called Blue Cranberries (or some variation) in the Carolinas. Western *Vacciniums* are much smaller plants—except for the California Huckleberry, which is larger and coarser—than the better known plants of the eastern states. California Huckleberry *(V. ovatum)* is an evergreen shrub from four to six feet in height, found along north slopes of the coastal ranges, sporadic from San Diego to Santa Barbara, common northwards. The leaves are leathery, alternate, with a deep indented center vein. The edges are finely toothed, the shape oval-lanceolate, and the color lighter underneath. The few terminal flowers are flesh colored and bell shaped, the berries succulent and edible though often bland, and dark purple to black but without the "bloom" of other species. Rocky Mountain Blueberry *(V. myrtillus* or *V. oreophilum* depending on the text) is a very different plant, smaller but more typical. It is a low, matting plant of a foot in height, forming large colonies in spruce forests above 8,000 feet in Arizona, New Mexico, and points north. The leaves are deciduous, oval-lanceolate, light translucent green, and form loose, open foliage interspersed with many short stems or branches. Between birds and small mammals the berries are seldom seen in any quantity, but they are purple and juicy, often found hanging from the underside of the branches. In high mountain roads the upward slopes can be covered with bright colonies of the plants. The steeper banks of high mountain creeks are a reliable starting place to look for our various, closely related Blueberries, with similar species found in all the higher ranges from the Sierra

37

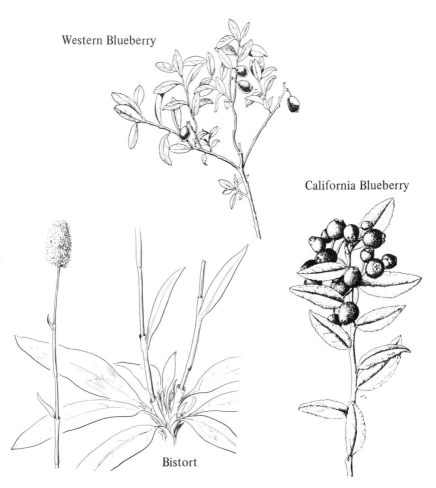

Western Blueberry

California Blueberry

Bistort

Nevadas of California eastwards. Although not listed in the texts, Blueberries can be found in the highest reaches of the San Bernardino Mountains, but well off the trails. All species are spring bloomers.

COLLECTING: The leaves, Method A. In the coastal species, strip the leaves; otherwise, use all the leaves and finely chopped stems.

MEDICINAL USE: The leaves have the same basic pharmacology as Uva Ursi, with rather less astringency, and may be used similarly. Further, they contain quinic acid, a former therapeutic for gout said to inhibit uric acid formation but never widely used because of mixed clinical results. Still, although certainly not as strong as standard medications, it is far less harmful and, like so many of the plants in this book, fills the void between health and acute disease. The leaves have been widely used to lower or modify blood sugar levels, particularly in Europe. Taken on a regular basis, two cups a day or one before dinner, Blueberry tea will gradually help alleviate both glycosuria and hyperglycemia and has a benign but useful effect as an adjunct treatment to diabetes mellitus.

BLUE CURLS

Trichostema spp.   Labiateae

OTHER NAMES: Wooly Blue Curls, Vinegar Weed, Romero (California Spanish)
APPEARANCE: Blue Curls are strongly scented members of the mint family, with erect, somewhat stiff or (in the perennials) woody stems, thin, lance-shaped leaves resembling rosemary, and sagelike terminal puffs of peculiarly shaped lavender to pink flowers, often densely woolly. The stamens protrude far out of the flowers, like insolent frog tongues. The foliage tends to be somewhat sticky, with a pleasant sweet-sour smell, and the overall height, especially in the more common perennial species, tends to run between two and three feet.
HABITAT: Common in the mountains of Los Angeles, Ventura, and Santa Barbara counties, as well as inland and northwards. *T. lanatum* is the commonest of the southern species, and ranges from San Diego to Monterey, between 2,000 and 4,000 feet, usually associated with Yerba Santa, White Sage, and buckwheat bush. Other varieties of only local abundance grow in the southern mountains of Arizona and New Mexico, usually on rocky slopes at about 6,000 feet.
COLLECTING: Flowering stems, Method A.
MEDICINAL USE: Most Blue Curls have a delicious sour-pine taste and make lovely herb tea, the flowering tops especially having a sweet aftertaste, altogether peculiar and delightful. A tea of the herb will settle a stomach ache as quickly as chamomile and promotes sweating in dry fevers. The tea is a mild menstrual stimulant and was used by the Chumash Indians to help expel the afterbirth in labor.

BLUE FLAG   (see color plate)

Iris missouriensis   Iridaceae

OTHER NAMES: Wild Iris, Western Blue Flag, Rocky Mountain Iris, Lirio (N.M.)
APPEARANCE: This is the predominant iris of the West, and in fact the only species native to our area outside of central California northwards. It is a typical iris, with long, smooth lance-shaped leaves, a light lavender to bluish purple flower slightly smaller than garden varieties. The plants form colonies and often cover whole meadows with their beautiful midsummer blossoms. The creeping rootstalk is reddish brown and covered with the leaf scales of previous growth. The true Blue Flag of herbal usage and other medicinal practice is *I. versicolor,* the common blue iris of gardens, and native to the eastern U.S.
HABITAT: Blue Flag is found in wet areas, moist meadows and the borders of sumps in all the mountains of our area that reach 8,000 feet, although in higher mountains with greater precipitation they may descend to as low as 5,500 feet. In California, stands are found only in the San Bernardino, San Jacinto, Mt. Pinos, and Sierra Nevada ranges, but they are common in all of the higher mountains of Arizona, New Mexico, and points north. The other irises of northern California and the Northwest may be useful but should be approached with caution. As in the internal uses of alternate species in general, the further the plants differ from the recognized varieties, the more unpredictable may be their effects, and even the feeblest iris can be toxic in immoderation.
COLLECTING: The creeping rootstalks, cleaned of the bulk of the dead chaff and dried on a flat surface. Pick in the fall or spring if possible.
MEDICINAL: At one time Blue Flag and its resin were the treatment of choice with physicians and eclectics that shared a revulsion for the more accepted (and highly

toxic) treatment of syphilis with bismuth, arsenic, mercury, and such. The main advantage of Blue Flag therapy was a lessened likelihood of poisoning the patient. It did help some individuals of particularly hardy constitution, but otherwise seemed to do little other than somewhat increase the natural defense mechanisms. More appropriately, the main effects of the drug are upon the digestive system and the secretory organs. Blue Flag was official for such purposes in the *National Formulary* until 1947, and is still widely used by English herbalists and the medical communities of other countries, particularly the Orient. The active principle is an oleoresin complex formerly called "iridin" and loosely classed with the phenol glycosides. Our species is actually more potent than the official plant and was formerly harvested for extraction.

The fresh roots are toxic and should not be used internally, but a poultice of the raw rhizome is especially effective against staph sores. Only the dry root should be tinctured. As a cathartic, two capsules of the ground root ("00" size) or twenty drops of the tincture is an average dose. The active principles are poorly water soluble, and capsules or tincture are preferable; nonetheless, one-fourth to one-half teaspoon of the chopped root, boiled in water for ten minutes, will serve as an energetic cathartic for most. It has a stimulating effect on the production of both pancreatic enzymes and bile. A single capsule between meals or with fresh vegetable or grapefruit juice and a three-day fast is an efficient way to make major dietary changes, particularly from a "pure" diet (that is, macrobiotic or vegan and the like) to one more broadly omnivorous. Whatever one's feeling about severely limited diets, if they are of long duration they should not be changed overnight; this little regimen will help facilitate such changes. A single capsule between meals is also useful where bile insufficiency results in poor oil absorption or periodic light-colored feces not directly related to drug therapy. Blue Flag was formerly used in treating jaundice, as its biliary effects cause a reflex stimulation of some liver functions; it is inadvisable for use in either chronic or acute liver malfunction or with drug therapies of a more serious nature.

Since the speed and mode of metabolization and excretion can be of critical importance in many substantial medical treatments, decreased or increased effects from such drugs may result from the accompanying use of Blue Flag. It is strong in effect and can be unpleasant if used in excess; therefore, its present use is almost always in combination with other herbs. As a stimulant to lymphatic function, it should be combined with Redroot or echinacea, one-half teaspoon of Blue Flag with two tablespoons of either, boiled for twenty minutes in a pint of water and drunk in small doses during the day. It is one of the traditional herbal alteratives, and can be combined with Burdock, Yellow Dock, Figwort, Inmortal, echinacea, sarsaparilla, gotu kola, and ginseng. Such combinations are useful in skin eruptions resulting from internal imbalances or blood toxicities, and especially when the condition involves an active infection or septicemia. Small, frequent doses of Blue Flag are a strong diuretic that has been used for various dropsies, and will also stimulate both saliva and sweat, further indicating its strong parasympathomimetic uses. This is a useful drug plant but in general should be used with care and preferably in combinations where less energetic plants form the bulk of a formula.

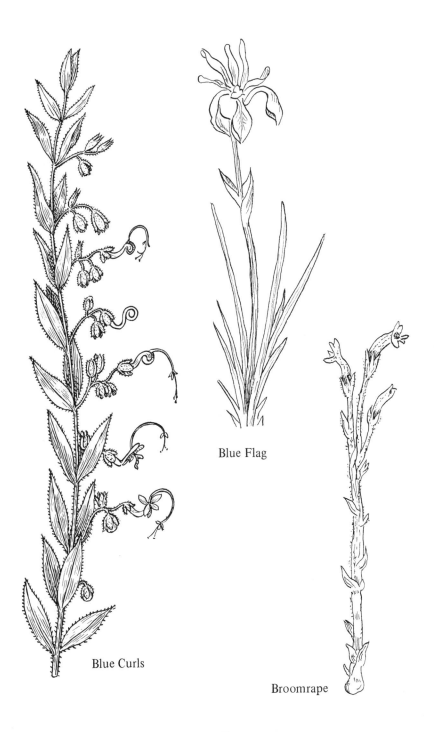

Blue Flag

Blue Curls

Broomrape

BROOMRAPE

(see color plate)

Orobanche spp.   Orobanchaceae

OTHER NAMES: *Epifagus, Epiphegus,* Beechdrops, Ghost Plant, Cancer Root

APPEARANCE: Broomrapes are weird. They are root parasites lacking chlorophyll, with a pale ghostlike appearance, the leaves having degenerated into scales, and the general color of the plants somewhere between puke white and butterscotch orange. The flowers vary from white to violet, forming either dense terminal spikes (in fact, most of the aboveground plant) or a pretty rosette of flowers at the end of the stalks. They are five lobed, two above that are parallel and three below that are spreading, with four stamens. Broomrape can be confused with the following parasites: Coral Root (thin and erect with widely spaced flowers that are orchidlike and usually three lobed with the roots bearing symbiotic molds and not attached to another plant); pine drops (the flowers bell-like with five little reflexed lobes); Snow Plant (thick and dark red). These are plants of the conifer forest only.

HABITAT: Widespread but peculiar and erratically unpredictable. Most Broomrapes are parasites of common shrubs, generally found between 3,000 and 6,000 feet. In Arizona, however, they may be found nearly to sea level and growing off cacti roots. The most common hosts are Sagebrush *(Artemisia tridentata),* Wild Buckwheat *(Eriogonum* sp.), Yerba Santa, Manzanita, Ragweed *(Ambrosia, Franseria),* and even Scrub Oak and Elder.

COLLECTING: Owing to the usual scarcity of Broomrape in any one area, it is always advisable to dig only one out of four visible plants, leaving the rest untouched. Although the root possesses the greatest activity, the whole plant is usable. Fortunately these plants usually strike down in loose soil, as the root (actually the below-ground stem) will descend from four inches to two feet, depending on the depth of the host root. If the host plant has several Broomrapes, dig only the plant(s) most distant from the host, thereby preserving the root sap for less distal Broomrapes. Dry as in Method B, preferably in an oven set at 160 degrees; like many fungi and parasitic plants, they putrify easily.

MEDICINAL USE: The whole plant is strongly astringent and makes an excellent poultice. Internally it is a mild laxative, sedative, and has been used to restore muscular strength and tone after debilitating illnesses and mild strokes. The whole family is highly prized in China as an aphrodisiac (probably due either to its relaxing effect or its ornately phallic appearance), and more recently has maintained a place in Chinese clinical treatments for menopausal hot flashes and as a confirmed uterine hemostatic. The average dose is a scant to rounded teaspoon boiled in water, one or two cups a day.

BUGLEWEED

Lycopus spp.   Labiateae

OTHER NAMES: Water Bugle, Water Horehound

APPEARANCE AND HABITAT: There are two species in the Southwest, *L. lucidus* and *L. americanus,* but, considering their intermingled habitat and crossbreeding, the difference is moot, although the first is slightly more astringent, the second slightly more sedative. Suffice it to say that Bugleweed is a typical member of the mint family, with square stems and opposing leaves. The flowers grow in axillary whorls of tiny pink or white flowers, frequently only on the leaf-bearing sides of the stems. Only Poleo and Motherwort share this axillary flower habit; Horehound and some Sages may share this configuration but not its wet habitat. Bugleweed is found almost solely along running water or in wet backwashes. *L. lucidus* has thick, round-cornered stems with leaves evenly, bluntly serrated and roots frequently bearing semituberous or noduled thickenings. *L. americanus* has more pronounced corners on the stems, smooth mintlike roots, and deeply cut, almost pinnate leaves. In California, Bugleweed is fairly abundant at lower altitudes, but in Arizona, New Mexico, and northwards it is a plant of the middle mountain areas and lower watersheds, abundant in the Rio Grande, Gila, Little Colorado, and Salt River basins along with their tributary streams and irrigation networks. Seldom encountered in high, isolated creeks, it should be looked for below 7,500 feet in cultivated or rural-suburban waterways.

COLLECTING: Method A.

MEDICINAL USE: Like Hops, Bugleweed is a specific for nervous indigestion, being both tonic and nervine. As a sedative or tranquilizer it is strong but not "druggy," producing few symptoms other than relaxation, larger doses causing pleasant, mild lethargy. For those individuals who resist sedatives and cling to their controlled stresses as a means of self-identity, this is much better than something like Valerian with its distinct, tactile drug effects. Bugleweed is a good hemostatic or coagulant for home use, nearly as specific as shepherd's purse without the latter's diuretic or hypertensive effects. As a rule it requires more frequent doses, however. The fresh tincture is preferable, but the dried herb is adequate; one-fourth to one-half teaspoon of the tincture or a rounded teaspoon to tablespoon of the herb in tea. Treatment should be continued one dose after the bleeding has stopped to allow firm clotting or sealing. It can be used for nosebleeds, excess menstruation, bleeding piles, and the like; Bugleweed is as effective as shepherd's purse for passive hemorrhage but not as effective as an emergency first aid. A cup every two or three hours as needed. Particularly useful for two or three days after labor, exerting little effect on colostrum or milk production.

BURDOCK

Arctium minus   Compositeae

OTHER NAMES: Clotbur, Lappa

APPEARANCE: Burdock is a large, coarse biennial, with huge, oval basal leaves, two feet or more in length, distinctly lighter below. The whole plant is rough textured, almost sandpapery. The first year's growth is a large rosette of irregular basal leaves, wrinkled and broadly undulating. In the second year a large thickly-leaved stalk appears in the center, forming many alternate branches and eventually reaching four or five feet in height and terminating in cherry-sized inconspicuous flowers, drab, bristly, and purple hued. These are densely thistlelike, with each bristle ending in a little back-hook. The purple flowers fade and the bristles stiffen into a more efficient burr without any change in actual shape, until in maturity the burr encloses a number of shiny dark seeds. Burdock is sometimes confused with Cocklebur *(Xanthium* spp.), a smaller, related annual having few basal leaves. The Cockleburs are little bristly capsules that grow in clusters along the stem, the two inner seeds resembling those of sunflowers when shelled. Conversely, Burdock burrs are chaffy and not at all solid, the seeds loosely bound within the chaff. The roots are carrotlike, fibrous, slightly aromatic, and from one to two feet long.

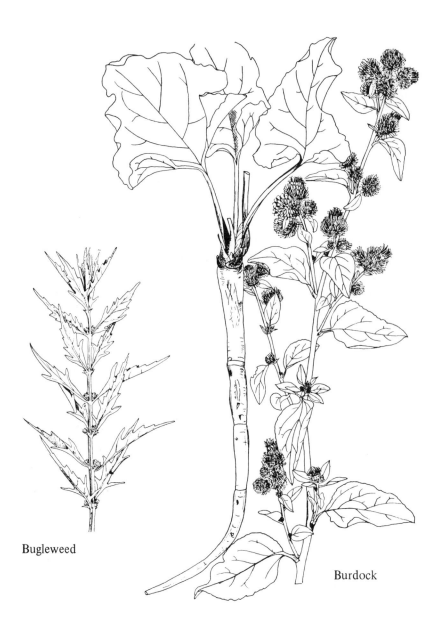

Bugleweed

Burdock

HABITAT: A European plant, Burdock is sporadic in our area; common in Idaho, Wyoming, Montana, Colorado, and northern New Mexico, occasional in Utah, Arizona, and Nevada, rare in southern California. Once established, Burdock becomes both common and hated, but may not be encountered again for fifty miles in any direction. Except for a few stands in the coastal ranges of California, in our area it is a plant of the middle altitudes, 5,000 to 8,000 feet. Burdock needs a fair amount of moisture and decent soil; it can be encountered in older farming and abandoned homestead areas. Livestock frequently spread the burrs as well as fertilizing the surrounding soil, and plants will often first establish in moist grazing areas because of this. Burdock can often be found in alluvial flats formed by descended mountain creeks. Still, you would be best served by checking your local herbarium for localities, particularly in California and Nevada. Although this will probably be private farming and grazing land, no sane rancher or farmer could possibly object to donating his or her Burdock stands.

COLLECTING: The seeds are picked in the fall after the burrs have lost any purple hue and turned drab brown. The seeds can be loosened from the chaff with a rolling pin or blender and winnowed. The roots, depending on which authority is consulted, should be dug in the fall of the first year or the spring of the second year, when first-year seedlings are just sprouting—my preference. Harvesting fully flowered plants in the fall can be as much work as digging a small tree; in addition to being covered top to bottom with the burrs, you will probably end up with a partially decayed root. Digging is best accomplished with a nurseryman's shovel, the long narrow type. Split and dry as in Method B.

MEDICINAL USE: Burdock is a widely used blood purifier and alterative, stronger than sarsaparilla but less energetic than echinacea and with little of the intestinal effects of Yellow Dock. Echinacea works best when dealing with an active infection or acute toxicity that results in skin eruptions; Yellow Dock is preferable when there are intestinal and liver malfunctions causing the toxicity; sarsaparilla is a more passive herb requiring other herbs for maximum effect and usually employed when gonad or adrenocortical secretions are causative; Burdock, however, works best when there are chronic and nonacute skin, sweat, or sebaceous eruptions, ranging from acne to psoriasis. An average regimen, which should be continued for at least two weeks, consists of a scant or rounded teaspoon in a cup of cold water, brought to a boil, simmered for twenty minutes, and drunk morning and evening. If the diuretic effects are too pronounced, the second cup may be drunk in late afternoon.

For any fast longer than three or four days, Burdock and Yellow Dock are useful adjuncts, helping to maintain peristalsis and prevent blood acidity and ketosis which usually accompanies overambitious fasting. The keratolytic (skin-softening) effects of a strong tea or the fresh root make it useful in treating keratosis pilaris. The seeds are an excellent diuretic, particularly for water retention and mild kidney-related toxemia—a half teaspoon boiled in water, two or three times a day as needed. In pregnancy the seeds may be used, but only in the last trimester and only in smaller quantities, with fifteen or twenty seeds per day in tea, drunk occasionally. For treating preeclampsia, particularly mild forms, this should be accompanied by frequent light sweating, preferably passively in a sauna, to help augment kidney function through perspiration. Although not an emmenagogue as such, the seeds may aggravate spotting in the earlier stages of pregnancy and should only be employed in the last trimester when needed, particularly when an inappropriate amount of ankle swelling is present and the preeclampsia mild enough that full eclampsia is unlikely. A tincture of the seeds, twenty to forty drops several times a day, is an old herbal remedy for single or joint inflammations of the extremities. If there is an active group of skin eruptions around the joint(s), a similar quantity of the root tincture should be used instead. The root tincture or tea is a folk remedy of long standing in England for a prolapsed uterus. As in most of the uses of Burdock, small frequent doses are the best method here, as well as lower potencies homeopathically, and it is most effective if the prolapse is recent or from childbirthing.

CULTIVATION: From seed, in rich, moist, but not necessarily well-drained soil. Burdock can become a dubious legacy in virgin areas, however.

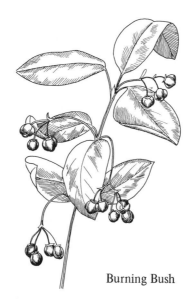

Burning Bush

BURNING BUSH
Euonymus occidentalis   Celastraceae

OTHER NAMES: Western Wahoo, Western Spindle Tree, Western Burning Bush

APPEARANCE AND HABITAT: Western Burning Bush or Wahoo is found only in the coastal states. A tall shrub or small tree, it ranges from six to twelve feet in height and has large, slightly triangular leaves two to four inches long, with green branches as far south as central California, whitish branches in Riverside and San Diego counties *(E. occidentalis, var. parishii)*. The flowers, three to seven, are borne on thin stems erupting from the axils of the opposing leaves. They are small, from one-fourth to one-half inch across, five petaled and purplish with the edges crisply reflexed. Seeds are small reddish capsules averaging one-fourth inch in length. With its square stems and opposing leaves, Burning Bush bears a passing resemblance to some large, diploid mint. In southern California, the variety is found only from the San Jacinto to Laguna Mountains, from 5,000 to 6,500 feet, although it may be looked for in the San Bernardino ranges. It is not encountered northwards until the Santa Cruz Mountains, then is common north to British Columbia and eastward to central Nevada.

COLLECTING: The bark of the larger stems and the roots, Method D.

MEDICINAL USE: A drug plant used in treating liver, gall bladder, and large intestine problems. May be used for liver "torpor" and constipation causing or resulting from poor bile secretion, particularly when evidenced by periodic light-colored feces that leave a slight oily film in water, lasting for a day or two and reoccurring from time to time. More specifically, in mild chronic cholecystitis without gallstones. It has been used in fevers resulting from liver inflammations, but the severity and cause should be judged by a physician first, since Burning Bush can overstimulate and aggravate more serious conditions. A scant teaspoon or less of the chopped bark is *steeped* for thirty minutes or more and drunk lukewarm. Wahoo is a mild cardiac stimulant for some, can manifest strong diuretic effects, and is a bronchial dilator and expectorant, but for whatever use some care is in order, as it has definite toxic potential in larger quantities.

CACHANA

Liatris punctata   Compositeae

OTHER NAMES: Blazing Star, Gayfeather, Rattlesnake Master

APPEARANCE: The leaves are long, slightly rough, and grasslike, crowded along the stems and intermingling with the lower flowers. The flower stalks can number from one to fifteen from a single root and are strikingly colored, ranging from violet pink to bluish purple. In the fall the flowers are replaced by dandelionlike seed puffs that are carried aloft by the wind. The root is pearly brown and nodular, ranging from a lumpy carrot to a round ball in shape. The inner pith is dark gray and slippery-starchy.

HABITAT: Eastern Wyoming and Colorado, central and northern New Mexico through the Texas Panhandle to the plains states. From 2,000 to 7,500 feet, generally along hillsides and road cuts in loose red dirt or gray clay.

COLLECTING: The roots in the fall after seeding. Method B. The flowers are best collected when partially in bud; otherwise, they will go to seed while drying and lose their color. Method A.

MEDICINAL USES: As a diuretic, to increase the volume of water in the urine for mild bladder and urethra infections and water retention. Of some use in decreasing phosphates in the urine if used for an extended period of time. Contains inulin, a starch that is not metabolized but is considered of use as a mild kidney and liver tonic by herbalists and used clinically to test kidney function. The root is also a useful tea for throat inflammation and laryngitis, a tablespoon of the chopped root boiled for twenty minutes in a cup of water and drunk slowly. A useful cough syrup can be made from equal volumes of the chopped fresh root and honey, mixed in a blender or macerated by hand, boiled slowly for one-half hour and strained. In New Mexico the rootlets are burned like incense and the smoke inhaled for headache and nosebleeds or blown into the throat for tonsil inflammations.

47

OTHER USES: The root has been used in a number of areas as a talisman and good luck charm. In the eastern and southern states a related species is called Rattlesnake Master and is supposed to ward off snakes and evil spells. In northern Mexico and New Mexico among both Hispanics and Indians, the root is carried or displayed as an artifact to ward off witches' spells and *mal de ojo* (evil eye), particularly to protect an infant. The round cormlike roots are sometimes split carefully in half and a crucifix carved in one half, the combined pieces then worn as a talisman.

CULTIVATION: The plant has a long flowering period and can be a striking addition to a garden. Best cultivated from freshly dug and transplanted roots, in either spring or late fall.

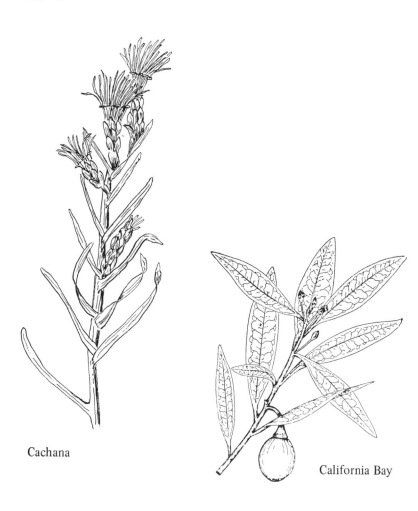

Cachana

California Bay

CALIFORNIA BAY

Umbellularia californica   Lauraceae

OTHER NAMES: California Laurel, Pepperwood Tree, California Pepper Tree, Oregon Myrtle, *Oreodaphne californica*

APPEARANCE: When mature, this is a tall, well-shaped tree of twenty to fifty feet in height, with many slender branches and bright shiny green oblong or lance-shaped leaves, strongly veined but relatively smooth. When crushed they give off a strong acrid-camphor smell that can be unpleasantly strong if inhaled for more than a moment. The evergreen leaves are smooth margined and alternate, very short petioled and two to four inches long. Small, young plants, sometimes little more than several floppy branches, have the same size leaves with the same potency as the largest majestic arboreal individuals with verdant, spreading crowns, touching the opposite walls of steep canyons. The flowers are tiny light green nothings, in little clusters of five to ten, ripening into purple-brown solitary drupes of an inch or less in size.

HABITAT: All the western ranges of California from San Diego northwards, through the Sierra Nevadas to southern Oregon, generally below 5,000 feet, reaching their greatest size in canyon bottoms and flood plains.

COLLECTING: Smaller, well-leaved branches, Method A, or larger branches dried singly. The dried leaves should be left intact.

MEDICINAL USE: The crushed leaves are an excellent herbal "smelling salt," held briefly under the nose of a person who is faint or has fainted. Prolonged breathing of the crushed leaves can cause a short-term frontal headache which can be cured, oddly enough, by a tea of the leaves. In general, the crushed leaves make an excellent tea for headache and neuralgia, possessing substantial anodyne effects, and they further have value as a treatment for the tenesmus or cramps from diarrhea, food poisoning, and gastroenteritis in general—two to four leaves crushed and steeped for tea, repeated as needed.

OTHER USES: The leaves are a substitute for bay laurel leaves from Europe (the traditional bay leaves) but must be used much more sparingly, since they can easily overpower a stew or soup. Unfortunately, they are often sold as regular bay leaves by commercial spice brands but without the warning to use less. The wood is excellent for lathe work and polishes beautifully.

CALIFORNIA POPPY

Eschscholtzia californica   Papaveraceae

APPEARANCE: This well-known wildflower grows from one to two feet tall, and has many finely, well-dissected basal leaves that are distinctly bluish in the spring. Unlike many of the poppy family, the sap is not milky. Although noted as a spring bloomer, in some areas the plant may flower until autumn. The flowers are four petaled and the color of orange sherbet, ripening into seed pods that are shaped like carpet needles with a little torus or ring around the base.

HABITAT: All sorts of places. In California it is found almost anywhere below 5,000 feet that has a slope and some moisture in the spring, usually west and south of the Sierra Nevadas, eastwards to the Mohave Desert. *E. mexicana,* considered by some to be identical with *E. californica,* is found periodically throughout Arizona, which is fortunate since it is illegal to pick the plant in California. Various intergrades are also found in New Mexico, Colorado, Utah, Texas, and Nevada. It is a common nursery plant with many varieties and hybrids; it often goes feral and can be found in the most surprising places below 7,000 feet. Although a perennial, it may become an annual in lower mountain meadows. It is difficult to miss with its large, showy yellow to orange red flowers.

COLLECTING: The whole aboveground plant, Method A.

MEDICINAL USE: Like so many of the family, a mild sedative and analgesic, suitable even for children. A rounded teaspoon of the chopped plant as tea. Excess quantities can cause a slight residual hangover the next morning. Note to would-be "Opium Eaters": The tea is functional, not fun.

CAÑAIGRE

Rumex hymenosepalus   Polygonaceae

OTHER NAMES: Red Dock, Pie Plant, Tanner's Dock, Wild Rhubarb

APPEARANCE: Cañaigre has thick, smooth, somewhat succulent leaves, one-half to one and one-half feet long, lance shaped, somewhat wavy with a pronounced central vein, and sour tasting. Leaves are mostly basal, trailing along the ground, with occasional alternate shorter leaves clasping the single stout stem, which grows from one to three feet tall. The top half of the stem bears many inconspicuous green flowers in the spring that mature into a thick, showy cluster of pink seed pods, three winged and somewhat heart shaped. The most definite identification comes from Cañaigre's underground cluster of yamlike tubers, from two to as many as a dozen. They are dark reddish brown with an inner flesh ranging from light orange to dark rust red, intensely astringent to the taste.

HABITAT: Surprisingly varied. It grows in luxuriance in the heart of the Mohave Desert and the dry mountains of eastern California and Arizona, the high plains of Utah and west Colorado to the eastern foothills of the Sangre de Cristo Mountains of New Mexico (7,000 feet), and throughout the great basin. The best plants for medicinal use tend to be found in and around dry sandy arroyos of the high desert, 3,000–5,000 feet, and dry mountain washes.

COLLECTING: Easier to dig if in elevated ground and sandy soil, difficult or impossible in gravelly basin sediment. Although very slow to rot, it is best to cut in one-fourth inch cross slices; a whole dried tuber can be a heavy, ugly, purposeless thing. The slices should be spread on paper and sun dried.

MEDICINAL USES: Like other docks, the root is rather complex biochemically, but so high in tannin as to make it useless for anything else. Prized by New Mexicans as a medicine, its relative Yellow Dock, although considerably lower in tannin levels, is shunned as being poisonous—because of its tannin! If you ever are sunburned to any degree in a desert area where both Cañaigre and any cactus are found, a not unlikely combination, the root can be grated fresh on the burned skin, allowed to dry, and a poultice of the inner pith of the cactus placed over or the juice rubbed in. The roots are boiled for an astringent and hemostatic wash for cuts and scrapes, or a mouthwash and gargle for ulcerations of the gums and mucosa, wherever astringency is needed. A final note: *Panax quinquefolium* (ginseng) and Cañaigre have nothing botanically or biochemically in common and have no similarities in function, habitat, appearance, or even taste. Cañaigre is a robust, rather common plant, whereas wild American ginseng is so rare as to be approaching $200.00 a pound wholesale. Since there are no legal standards to the "Ginseng" name,

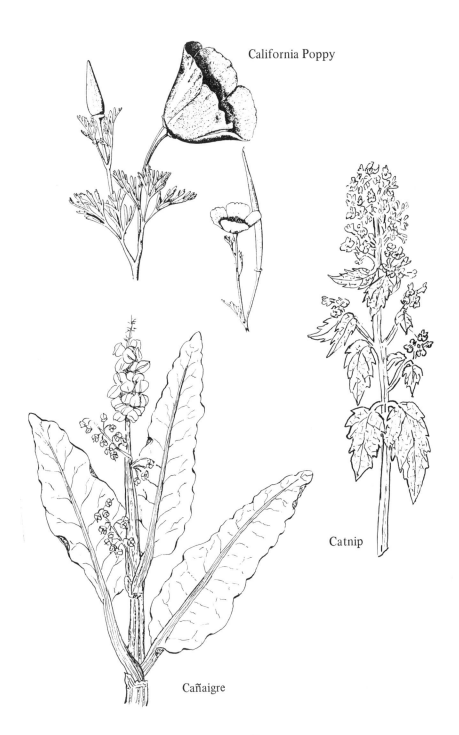

California Poppy

Catnip

Cañaigre

several companies are marketing Cañaigre, grossly overpriced, as "Wild Red Desert Ginseng," capitalizing on the expense of true wild ginseng, the reddish color of some grades of *cured* oriental ginseng, and the lack of knowledge on the parts of some health food stores and the public.

OTHER USES: The leaves can be used as a substitute for rhubarb.

CATNIP

Nepeta cataria   Labiateae

APPEARANCE: Catnip has the usual square stem and opposing leaves of the mint family; its average height is from two to three feet, but along creek banks and ditches in comely locations it may approach the improbable altitude of five feet. The flowers appear in Sage-like terminal clusters, white or light pink with violet or purple markings. Leaves are somewhat triangular with roundly serrated edges. The whole plant is densely downy like fine felt, with a distinctly grayish color under moist root but full sun locations. For those of you who have never grown Catnip but have only come in contact with it as an herb tea or cat intoxicant, the smell of fresh or reasonably recent dried Catnip is strong, minty, with a slightly rank after-smell. If you must buy it, crush a little between your fingers; if there is no smell, ignore it. It's only fit for the most addicted feline. Good Catnip, however, will drive the little carnivores into an almost indecent frenzy. If your cat is controlled, indifferent, prissy-efficient, and gives you an inferiority complex, a few fresh leaves will remove all inhibitions. The animal will grovel, drool, and make a benign fool of itself. Oriental cats sometimes find this beneath them.

HABITAT: In our area Catnip is a mountain plant. It is found infrequently in the southern half of California, generally in moist developed mountain valleys such as Lake Arrowhead and above Ojai and the like. In Arizona north of the Mogollon Rim and around Flagstaff and sporadically in the mountains around Tucson and Phoenix. Catnip is encountered with some regularity above 6,500 feet in moist resort areas and population centers. Common around people throughout the Rockies from the Manzanos (New Mexico) northwards, at least where there is substantial forestation, and found sometimes in nearly virgin land. Even here, however, an abandoned summer cabin or logger's station is probably not far away.

COLLECTING: The whole green plant, Method A. In some localities, Catnip can be a very substantial plant, with thick, almost woody stems; these should be removed or used for tincturing. If you have a coldly practical nature, save them for your cats.

MEDICINAL USES: A mild but reliable tranquilizer and sedative. It will not faze serious insomnia or the terminal hypers, but the tea is gentle, sure, and safe even for children and infants. It is an excellent colic tea or teething tea; a tincture of fresh Catnip with an equal weight of fennel seed in four times their total volume of vodka is a very effective treatment for indigestion, stomach aches, and hiccups, one-fourth to one-half teaspoon in water. Catnip has a mild antispasmodic effect and may be used for cramps, but it may act to increase menstrual flow to varying degrees. Technically, Catnip, like chamomile, should probably not be used in pregnancy for this reason, but the chances of stimulating spotting are remote.

CULTIVATION: The seeds in spring, planted in fairly moist, fairly decent soil. According to Grieve, the seeds will still germinate after five years. In lower altitudes of the West, Catnip will need a fair amount of watering; more than Horehound, less than the true mints.

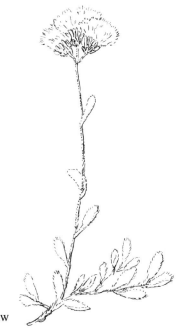

Cat's Paw

CAT'S PAW

Antennaria spp.   Compositeae

OTHER NAMES: Pussy-Toes, Life Everlasting, Mountain Everlasting, etc.

APPEARANCE: This is a plant that forms densely hairy little mats of basal rosettes and four- to six-inch flower stalks. The little mats are distinctly silvery gray; the flowers are small pearly buttons clustered around the top of the hairy stem, forming a fair approximation of the underside of a kitten's paw, with colors ranging from pearly gray to pink in higher altitudes. The basal leaves remind me, in their ground-hugging, pointed-oval symmetry, of the stylized foliage found on silver serving ware made in the last century.

HABITAT: Found throughout the mountains of the West, generally in substantial forests, from just above the Ponderosa or Yellow Pine belt to timberline. A common plant among major stands of pine and spruce, growing in the rocky areas above the needle mulch.

COLLECTING: The whole blooming plant, rootlet, basal leaves, and flowering stalklets. If not overly moist when picked, they may be dried loosely in a paper bag or box, but if taken from high, moist mountains, Method C.

MEDICINAL USE: As daintily useless as it may appear, Cat's Paw is an excellent remedy for liver inflammation and a mild recurrence of former hepatitis symptoms—a tablespoon of the chopped plant steeped in water. It is also a good nonirritating astringent for intestinal irritations above the ileocecal valve. By the time the colon is reached its effect is nil, so should be used as an enema if needed for the descending colon or rectum. The tea is a useful douche for vaginitis.

CEBADILLA

Swertia radiata   Gentianaceae

OTHER NAMES: Green Gentian, American Columbo, Deer's Ears, *Frasera speciosa*

APPEARANCE: A distinctly two-formed plant, either biennial or triennial. The first stage is a large rosette of lilylike leaves, radiating gracefully out from·the center, with leaves a foot or two in length and oval to lance-shaped. The whole plant is waxy smooth. In the flowering stage the plant may reach six feet in height and is conspicuous when encountered. The single upright stalk arises from the center of the basal leaves and is covered with whorls of attractive greenish flowers with a rosette of four to six thin leaves beneath. The plant nearly always dies after seeding, casting about tiny dark seeds.

HABITAT: Very rich, very moist forest, most commonly on mild slopes, from 7,000 to 10,000 feet in our highest ranges. Always in partial shade, Cebadilla may grow in small stands or with solitary widespread plants interspersed throughout the forest. Not a common plant, it is frequent enough to list here.

COLLECTING: The yellow root of the unflowered plant, generally in the fall. Method B. The roots of flowering plants are already beginning to rot by autumn and are unusable. The fresh roots are not used.

MEDICINAL USES: Primarily a medicine for the digestive tract. Similar to Gentian in its effect, it is more energetic and irritating. A stimulant to stomach and small intestinal secretions and contractions, it makes a bitter tonic especially useful for the elderly. The dried root is powdered, six to eight tablespoons added to a pint of brandy, and it is steeped for at least a week; a tablespoon is taken before meals. A pinch of the powder in sweetened water has a similar effect. One-half to one teaspoon of the root powder boiled in water will act as a laxative-cathartic. More than a teaspoon can act as an irritant to the large intestine, and in any respect Cebadilla should be used as a laxative only occasionally. The root can also serve as a fungicide for athlete's foot, jock rot, and the like. Sometimes effective as a tincture for ringworm, but care should be taken; when used on children it can irritate the skin. In New Mexico the powdered root is melted in lard and applied on the scalp to kill lice or rubbed on the legs to kill scabies. I have never talked to anybody who has done this and have no idea of how effective it is . . . it does sound messy, though.

CULTIVATION: Probably difficult, but could be attempted if the seeds are frozen several times while in peat and sown in early spring in very rich soil. It might take up to two years for some to germinate, so be patient.

CHICORY   (see color plate)

Cichorium intybus   Compositeae

APPEARANCE: A scruffy, weedy plant, with many two- or three-foot sticklike stems, open, widely spaced foliage, and milky sap. The striking thing about Chicory, however, is its bright, almost iridescent blue flowers that bloom incongruously on the stems as if stapled to the wrong plant.

HABITAT: Varied and unpredictable, ranging from a median strip between lanes on Olympic Boulevard in Santa Monica, California, to a high grazing pasture at 9,300 feet above Durango, Colorado. In the West, however, it is generally a mountain or

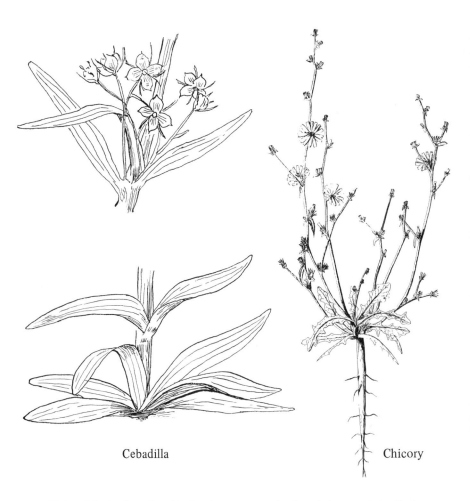

Cebadilla

Chicory

higher altitude plant, found in farming or pasture lands and along roads in all of our states.

COLLECTING: The light-colored taproots of spring, second-year plants, previous to any substantial flowering. Method B.

MEDICINAL: Identical with Dandelion but slightly weaker.

OTHER USES: Unlike Dandelion, Chicory makes a good coffee substitute. The roots, chopped sideways and completely dried, are roasted on a cookie sheet at 350 degrees until medium dark brown, cooled, and finely ground in a coffee mill or blender. When harvesting for roasting, it is especially important to pick before flowering, as the roots become progressively bitter as the growing season wears on. If mixed with coffee, use two parts coffee and one part roasted chicory, decreasing the total grounds by one-third.

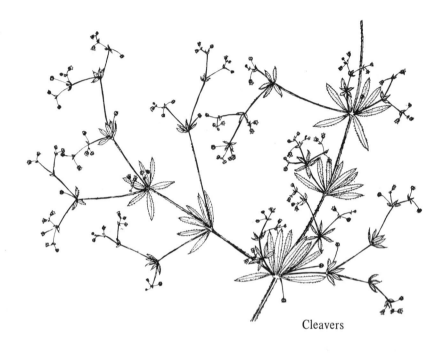

Cleavers

CLEAVERS

Gallium aparine   Rubiaceae

OTHER NAMES: Cleaver's Wort, Goosegrass, Clivers, Bedstraw, Catchweed Bedstraw

APPEARANCE: There are many species of *Gallium* in the West, but Cleavers is by far the most common variety. This is a naturalized annual, in contrast with the predominantly perennial native *Galliums*. These latter, which are often loosely called bedstraws, form a large group of less common plants; the difference is moot, since both Cleavers and the natives are all used rather interchangeably and all have similar, if not identical, properties. Cleavers, with its single stem and square, bristly edges, most frequently forms little vinelike mats over and through taller herbs and shrubs. Larger plants might attain a length of six or seven feet if their many angular little branches could be unhooked and untangled, but all grows from a single weak stem starting somewhere behind or below the shrubbery. Native *Galliums* are either little shrublike clumps of stems or share a certain degree of the piggyback habits of Cleavers and may be smooth stemmed or bristly, but none are as successful as this intruder. All *Galliums* have square stems, and the foliage forms regular whorls of leaves along these stems. The leaves of Cleavers, roundly lanceolate, form circular rosettes of six or eight leaves; the bedstraws most frequently have only four leaves in a whorl. The flowers are white as a rule, and star shaped, either loose and open as in Cleavers or rather dense and lacy clusters in most of the native plants. The seeds of Cleavers are a bit peculiar, always in pairs and covered with little bristly hairs like green testicles. They turn brown in the fall. If no plants are convenient to grow upon, Cleavers and the climbing varieties of bedstraws will grow a few inches and start to form dense mats. In this growing habit they may be confused with carpetweed or *Mollugo,* a little round-stemmed plant with similarly whorled leaves that always grows in this fashion but has no medicinal value and, in fact, is completely unrelated.

HABITAT: Cleavers, a European native, is found in sheltered, fairly moist places from sea level to almost 10,000 feet, but in our area it is primarily a mountain plant. It frequents streamside shrubs, moist embankments, pastures, fence rows, and shady areas under trees. Other *Galliums,* although a bit more varied in habitat, are more likely to be found in similar circumstances. As they are mostly perennials, they may be found in somewhat drier and more exposed terrain. The genera, and particularly Cleavers, is found in all of our ranges.

COLLECTING: If it is a clinging bedstraw, it can simply be wadded up in loose mats and hung to dry or laid out to dry in the shade. Smooth-stemmed varieties may need to be bundled, Method A.

MEDICINAL USE: Cleavers (as well as all bedstraws) is used almost entirely in treating problems of the urinary tract and skin. Cleavers tea, itself a pleasant beverage, is a moderate but persistant diuretic, and useful in cases where such is needed. It has feeble effects on liver function but is one of the few herbs that has some healing value and yet may be used during hepatitis without fear of irritation. Due to this feebleness in usual tea doses, it may be used in more concentrated amounts to relieve inflammations of the lower urinary tract that result in painful urination and chronic dysuria. A tablespoon of the dried plant is made into tea and drunk three times a day an hour before meals. In cases of urinary calculi or gravel the tea is useful in the same manner, but the fresh plant is considerably more effective. Two to three teaspoons of the juice is drunk in a cup of water three times a day. It may be preserved by adding ten percent grain alcohol or twenty-five percent vodka or simply frozen and defrosted as needed. Since there is enough alcohol in this form of preserving to make some people a bit tipsy, teetotalers with a chronic recurring problem of this nature may prefer the freezing method; ice cube trays or (for those with a strong sense of the absurd) Popsicle freezing trays make it easier to defrost small quantities at a time. The juice or a strong tea is good for bathing slowly healing burns, ulcerated skin, inflamed stretch marks, or any suppurating skin conditions. The value of the fluid extract in physiological doses for suspending or modifying cancerous ulcers has had substantial clinical proving by homeopaths.

OTHER USES: The small roots, particularly of the perennial bedstraws, contain a pigment also found in madder, a close relative, and they can be used in a similar way for dyeing. The small seeds can be dried and roasted, English country style, to make a coffee substitute.

CULTIVATION: The seeds grow easily and can make an attractive ground cover in moist shady areas or when planted below shrubbery for a gossamer, viney effect. Self-seeding but prone to spreading out of control.

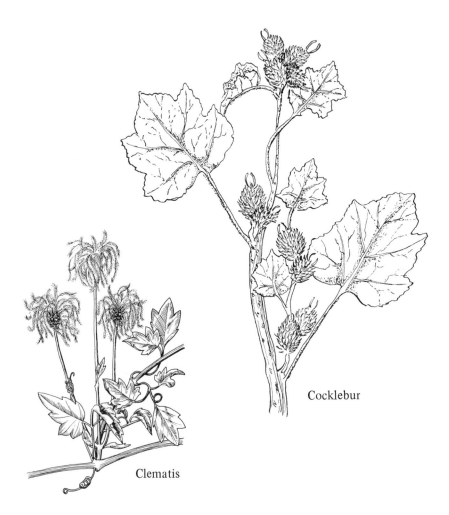

Cocklebur

Clematis

CLEMATIS   (see color plate)

Clematis spp.   Ranunculaceae

OTHER NAMES: Virgin's Bower, Western Virgin's Bower, Old Man's Beard, Barbo de Chivo

APPEARANCE: This is the most common vine in our mountains, with opposite leaves that are formed by three to seven stemmed leaflets and underlying tendrils for grasping. The two basic forms of flowers are quite dissimilar. One type has small cream-colored blossoms in dense clusters, the other has solitary downturned four-petaled flowers which are showy and mauve to purple. Either type of Clematis flower matures into a colony of long, silky plumes, recognizable in the fall. Most of our species are climbers, often forming vines forty feet or longer across the crowns of trees; some, however, form little scraggly semiupright clumps if nothing is available to climb on, or trail vaguely along the ground looking for a trunk.

HABITAT: Nearly everywhere above 4,000 feet, and especially in main forest areas. Often found in suburban areas around our higher towns and cities, but seldom above 8,500 feet.

COLLECTING: The long trailing branches, tied into bundles and finely chopped, stem and all, after drying. The less common purple-flower species is a bit stronger, but all are useful.

MEDICINAL USE: A tablespoon of the plant in tea seems to have a vasoconstrictor effect on the brain lining but a dilating effect on the veins. It is, therefore, a useful treatment for headaches in general and migraine and cluster headaches specifically. Although not reliable, it has worked where narcotics and ergot alkaloids have not helped and, considering the debilitating nature of these two problems, it is worth trying. Most effective in classic migraines where there are head flushes or visual disturbances in advance of the actual headache and most effective then, when drunk at the first sign of these presymptoms. Further, Clematis can increase the effectiveness of other therapies, either herbal or drug, and, as is so often the case with herbal remedies, seems to work better each time it is used. A tincture of the fresh plant is a useful counterirritant.

COCKLEBUR

Xanthium strumarium   Compositeae

OTHER NAMES: Cadillos, *X. canadense*

APPEARANCE: By nearly all standards this is a reprehensible, useless, and unpleasant weed lacking in any redeeming values. It is a widespread immigrant from the eastern states, growing to two feet in height, with large, rough three-lobed leaves with long stems which attain an overall length of as much as four or five inches in favoured locations. In mature plants the foliage is predominantly along the upper half of the main stem. The fruit is the ever-so-familiar cocklebur, the bane of hikers, pet owners, and sheepherders. Cockleburs are an inch long, egg-shaped, and covered with efficient recurved barbs. They cluster around the upper part of the stem and contain two nutlets about the size of shelled sunflower seeds.

HABITAT: Everywhere, but especially common and potent around the alluvial washes and creek banks of our mountains and upper foothills. They are frequently encountered in close-mouthed dried sumps.

COLLECTING: The burrs (with gloves) when ripe and brownish, dried loosely in paper bags or on newspapers. The leaving tops, Method A.

MEDICINAL USE: A tea of the leaves is a useful diuretic and is especially useful for chronic cystitis; a rounded teaspoon of the chopped leaves in tea, morning and afternoon. The seeds contain the glycoside xanthostrumarin and the germicide xanthatin. Three or four pods boiled in water will stop the most obstinate diarrhea. A teaspoon of the crushed pods boiled for five minutes has analgesic, diuretic, and antispasmodic effects, and has been used in many areas for rheumatism and arthritis. Cocklebur is not a completely benign herb, and large quantities or constant use can have toxic effects, particularly on the intestinal tract and liver. A tincture of the crushed seeds is both clotting and antiseptic for skin abrasions, and is a good first aid dressing.

CULTIVATION: Avoid at all cost.

COFFEE BERRY

Rhamnus californica   Rhamnaceae

OTHER NAMES: California Buckthorn, Pigeon Berry

APPEARANCE: A large shrub from four to ten feet in height, although individuals exceeding twenty feet and more properly termed trees may be encountered in Arizona. It has alternate leaves which are somewhat sparsely spaced on the branches and possess single, recessed center veins that give them a double concave form. The leaf edges vary widely from smooth to serrated but are usually narrowly oblong and from one and one-half to two and one-half inches in length. Like its relative Red Root, Coffee Berry forms endless varieties from range to range, and leaves may be broader or narrower, distinctly yellow on both sides or, particularly in Arizona and New Mexico, only underneath, and either smooth or finely hairy. The flowers are insignificant and green, star-shaped with five-pointed petals and stamens, and either semiclosed and budlike or fully opened. The seeds, at first green, become reddish and finally the color of roasted coffee . . . hence the name.

HABITAT: Frequent in California from San Diego County northwards, below 4,000 feet in the coastal ranges on open slopes, foothills, and canyons, often nearly to the beaches; eastward at higher elevations, sometimes above 6,500 feet, through all the ranges of Arizona and New Mexico. In Utah, Colorado, and northern New Mexico Coffee Berry intergrades with *R. smithii,* a four-petaled species of the Chaparral and Ponderosa belts.

COLLECTING: The bark of larger stems and younger trunks, Method D. *After* drying it is important to heat the bark for two days in an oven set at 110–120 degrees; otherwise the drug is strongly emetic and irritating to the intestinal tract.

MEDICINAL USE: Like its close relative cascara sagrada *(R. purshiana),* Coffee Berry is a laxative, containing emodin and other rhamnoid glycosides; a teaspoon of the chopped bark boiled for ten minutes is a starting dose, increased or decreased at a later date depending on its effects, which vary in different localities and varieties. Coffee Berry is especially useful for inflammatory rheumatism, where the joints are swollen and painful (Boericke)—a tablespoon of the bark boiled in an appropriate amount of water and drunk in four doses throughout the day. It is a mild liver stimulant and will increase bile secretions, primarily from the hepatic duct, less so for the gall bladder. On the other hand, some authorities consider the *rhamnus* barks to be a bile mimic, with little or no direct effect on the secretory functions at all. I am inclined to agree with the first position, but take your choice.

CONEFLOWER   (see color plate)

Rudbeckia hirta, R. laciniata   Compositeae

OTHER NAMES: Lance-Leafed Coneflower, Black-Eyed Susan, Golden Glow, Dormilón

APPEARANCE AND HABITAT: *R. laciniata* is a tall two- to four-foot perennial, found in the rich-soiled mountains of Arizona, Nevada, Wyoming, New Mexico, Utah, and Colorado, along streams and wet areas from 6,000 to 8,500 feet. The green stems bear cutleaf, variably shaped leaves, vaguely palmate when basal, gradually becoming simpler towards the terminal large yellow flowers. These are typical members of the aster family, with many somewhat irregular ray flowers and a large yellow cone of disc flowers, lightly flecked (in some areas) with brown. *R.*

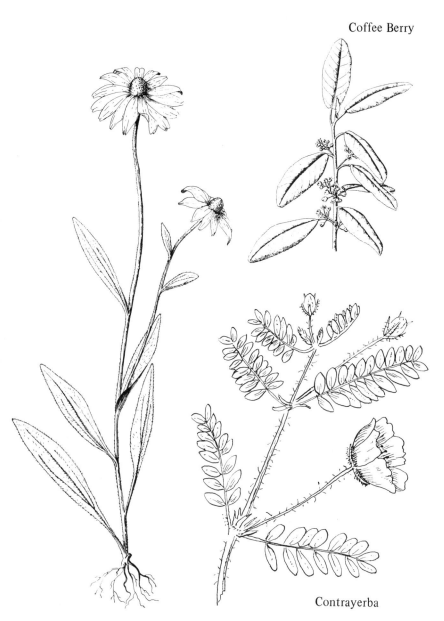

Coffee Berry

Coneflower (Black-Eyed Susan)

Contrayerba

hirta or Black-Eyed Susan is found in Colorado, New Mexico, Texas, northward and eastward. It is one to three feet tall, densely, almost irritatingly hairy, the leaves sometimes bearing little glandular purple dots, the lower leaves two to four inches long and oblong, becoming smaller and lanceolate towards the terminal flowers. These are yellow petaled with a dark brown cone of disc flowers. Both species have far less conical centers than the typical Coneflowers of the eastern states.

COLLECTING: *R. laciniata,* the root, Method B. *R. hirta,* the herb, Method A.

MEDICINAL USE: Both plants are stimulating diuretics, with feeble cardiac stimulation as a side effect. They can be relied upon to stimulate the volume of water but not the solids in the urine. The root or leaves, a teaspoon or more in tea as needed. The tea of the aboveground parts of *R. hirta* should be strained through a cloth to remove the hairs. The root of *R. laciniata* has a history of use for painful menstruation in New Mexico.

CONTRAYERBA   (see color plate)

Kallstroemia spp.   Zygophyllaceae

OTHER NAMES: Arizona Poppy, Mexican Poppy

APPEARANCE AND HABITAT: This is a ground cover plant, usually annual, with many hairy, prostrate stems covered with pinnate leaves, the whole sometimes having a circumference of several feet. The plant bears many pretty orange or yellowish orange poppylike flowers, usually in late summer or early fall. Contrayerba bears a close resemblance to its relative puncture vine (*Tribulus terrestrias*), the latter the source of those abominable little triangular spiked seeds that debilitate livestock, bare feet, and bicycle tires. The root is thin and insignificant, and this plant should not be confused with Contrayerba Blanca, an important *remedio* in Mexico (a flat oval white root), or Contrayerva, a medicinal plant from Central and South America (reddish brown, long, and wrinkled). The various species of *Kallstroemia* are frequent in the Mohave and Colorado deserts below 3,000 feet, and in Arizona, New Mexico, and Colorado to 6,000 feet on drier plateaus, mesas, and along roadsides and ditches. Will bloom at any time after late spring, following thunderstorms or substantial rain.

COLLECTING: The whole plant in bloom, Method A or C, depending on the size of the plants.

MEDICINAL USES: This Contrayerba is an effective astringent and hemostatic, with its effects lasting the length of the intestinal tract and therefore of use in dysentery and general intestinal inflammations. A tablespoon of the chopped plant is steeped in tea and drunk as needed. It may be used as a systemic hemostatic; when drunk after a sprain or major bruise or hematoma will help stabilize the injury and facilitate quicker healing. The tea will also lessen menstrual flow. A few leaves in a little water or a weak tea is a soothing eyewash.

CORAL ROOT (see color plate)

Corallorhiza maculata   Orchidaceae

OTHER NAMES: Crawley

APPEARANCE: This is an exotic little saprophytic orchid, lacking chlorophyll and having a light orange to brownish color. The leaves are reduced to a few sheathing scales, but it is otherwise naked-stemmed below the flowers and seldom reaches a foot in height. The flowers are brownish purple with dark flecks and, though small, are distinctly orchidlike, having a single spotted lower lip, two side-spurs, two upper petals, and another upright spur behind the blossom. They are in loose panicles that mature into little oval, drooping fruit.

HABITAT: A plant found frequently but always in small amounts in and above the Ponderosa belt, usually in shady thickets or modest slopes in well-forested areas. It is basically parasitic or symbiotic upon several species of molds that dwell in conifer and particularly Pine mulch, and may be found interspersed from San Diego County north and east, and throughout the United States, Canada, and Mexico; always, in our area, in main forest environments. Never common or numerous, it can still form stands of a dozen or more plants, and if one is encountered, several more are likely to be in the immediate vicinity. Like most parasitic plants, it is seldom found in direct sunlight or well-traveled areas. A single footstep will kill the aboveground growth until the following year; consequently, Coral Root is not often found by campsites or well-traveled trails although, after Mistletoe, it is the most common of our stranger plants.

COLLECTING: Only dig one of four visible plants; although widespread it does not propagate easily, and an overeager "picker" can plunder and pillage a whole watershed if care is not taken. The gray convoluted roots resemble coral growths or mutant brains, and are usually found at least six inches below the top of the needle mulch. A shovel should be used for digging, since the various invaginations of the root can break off into little pebble-like pieces if spaded or lifted up and are easily lost in the mulch. The whole clump should be carried in a bag until washed, and then rinsed under water in a sieve, the dirt removed at that time. The root should be rubbed into small pieces and allowed to dry on a newspaper or as in Method C as soon as possible to prevent the accompanying mold spores from causing spoilage.

MEDICINAL USE: Coral Root is one of the best treatments for nervous disorders and nervous fevers, a scant teaspoon boiled for ten minutes. It will reduce a fever reliably and has a strong, sensible sedative effect particularly useful for angry or frustrated states. It is especially good as a first aid for sudden high fevers in the first week or two after childbirth, usually caused by dehydration or (more important) a uterine infection. This is *not* a condition for home treatment, but Coral Root will relax the mother and lower the temperature until a physician can apply more appropriate therapies. It should be made available if needed for any rural-type home delivery. Such sudden fevers, although uncommon, can be devastating.

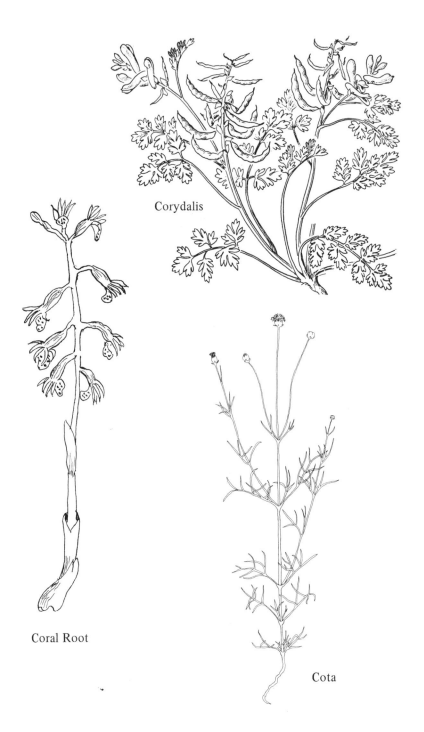

Corydalis

Coral Root

Cota

CORYDALIS

Corydalis aurea   Fumariaceae (Papaveraceae)

OTHER NAMES: Golden Smoke

APPEARANCE: This little clumpy plant has many spreading, slightly succulent stems radiating from a small rootstalk, and is covered with small, dissected leaves of a bluish green or bluish gray color. The flowers form little erratic racemes of yellow color and have a peculiar, vaguely pealike two-lobed form. Upon closer examination these flowers are atypical—angular, slightly inflated, and irregular. They mature into long beanlike pods that may be mixed helter-skelter with flowers in all other stages of development. Although rarely more than a foot tall, Corydalis is one of the first flowering plants in spring and one of the last to bloom in the fall. Often found in stands, but solitary plants are also common.

HABITAT: Arizona, New Mexico, and northwards, in a variety of circumstances, anywhere from 2,000 to 10,500 feet but most frequently in the main forest areas, Ponderosa, and above. Can be encountered along old cuts, roads, mine tailings, ski lodges, and new burn areas; not at all averse to human habitation.

COLLECTING: The whole plant, roots and foliage. Method A or C, depending on length of stems.

MEDICINAL USE: A member of one of two interrelated genera, *Dicentra* and *Corydalis,* both with complex, almost tortuous pharmacology. This species, the most common in the West, contains at least ten alkaloids, including corydaline, corypalmine, and protopine, but may or may not contain bulbocapnine, the only alkaloid from the two generas presently used in medicine. What all this means is that one-half teaspoon of the plant combined with a more specific herbal sedative such as Skullcap or Valerian will aid nervousness or hysteria that is manifest through trembling, shaking, twitching, or tics. It is not recommended in larger doses since it may cause these very same symptoms. Although neither strong nor safe alone, it is very effective in combination. The several species of *Dicentra* found in California may have similar effects but then again can be downright dangerous and are not advisable for herbal usage.

COTA

Thelesperma spp.   Compositeae

OTHER NAMES: Navajo Tea, Indian Tea, Colorado Green Thread, Té de Cota

APPEARANCE: A graceful plant from one to two feet in height with thin nodding stems and threadlike pairs of divided leaves widely spaced along the stems. The foliage is distinctly blue green and glaucous. Flowering from July to September, Cota is almost impossible to identify until it's in bloom. Several other plants bear superficial resemblance to it before flowering, but the taste of the leaves is intensely bitter, whereas Cota has a pleasantly piney sweet taste. The little gold tufted flowers are generally about the size of a nickel. Like other members of the Compositeae family, the "flower" is actually a colony of flowers, all without petals. They puff out from a waxy cuplike calyx that often becomes somewhat translucent brown with age. Once found, stands of Cota are distinctive, with the hundreds of gracefully nodding gold tufts contrasting with the blue green foliage below. The taste of the plant makes Cota one of our very best wild teas, and it is widely known in areas where it grows. Each plant has a small tan taproot with from one to a dozen stems branching from it. Some related species have small gold daisylike petals but most of our Cota is petalless.

HABITAT: From Arizona through to Texas and the plains states, and Colorado, Wyoming, and Utah. From 3,500 to 8,000 feet, frequenting roadsides, open meadows, and the lips of arroyos. Erratic in distribution, it may miss one county and inundate another. Back roads and low foothills in midsummer in medium-dry areas are good starting places.

COLLECTING: Method A.

MEDICINAL USE: A mild diuretic, useful in water retention and urethra irritations. Cota is mildly antiseptic to the urinary tract. Not a strong remedy, it can be useful because of its lovely taste. It makes a cooling summer ice tea, with some Spearmint and *piloncillo* (Mexican cone sugar). Like Spearmint, it is a good tea for convalescence, also useful for indigestion and mild fever. For the inveterate tea drinker, Cota can be positively addicting; along with Poleo and Mormon Tea, it is one of our three best native teas, a reddish beverage with distinctive aroma and flavor. It is a traditional beverage of many Spanish New Mexicans, as well as a widely used folk remedy for arthritis, kidney, and blood complaints. It is used with malva (*Malva neglecta*) as a skin wash for diaper rash and thrush. Among the Pueblo Indians its use is ancient; Cota twigs were even found with pottery shards in Chaco Canyon.

CULTIVATION: The mature, dark seeds are sown in the fall and covered with one-fourth inch of fine dirt. Taproots can be planted in the fall after the stalks have died down. Cota needs sunlight and good drainage. It is a good border plant for planting around roadways and walkways.

COW PARSNIP (see color plate)
Heracleum lanatum   Umbelliferae

OTHER NAMES: Cow Cabbage, American Masterwort, Yerba del Oso, Wooly Parsnip, *H. sphondylium*

APPEARANCE: This is a big, hairy, coarse member of the parsley family, as tall as five feet in height, with large, flat-topped umbels of white flowers. These flowers, sometimes forming heads a foot across, mature into large, flat seeds, round and deeply grooved. The stems are hollow, a family characteristic, and the root is large, light colored, and strong scented with a slightly soapy inner pith. The whole plant has a strong acrid-celery scent, nearly unbearable to the taste, particularly in the root and seeds, with a persistent numbing aftersensation. The large leaves may or may not be dissected and are either irregularly palmate or distinctly three leaved, the thick stems clasping an even thicker stalk that may reach two inches around. This is a large, conspicuous, pleasantly gross plant that is easily identifiable.

HABITAT: In California it is common in the higher coastal ranges, usually in or near water, and above 6,000 feet in the inner mountains and Sierra Nevadas. It is frequent in the middle elevations of the forests of California, Arizona, Nevada, Idaho, Utah, Colorado, Wyoming, Montana, and New Mexico, also in or near water. Above 8,500 feet it becomes common in moist meadows and wet hillsides away from water.

COLLECTING: The roots in late August or September, the seeds when ripe and ribbed with darker stripes, July or August. Roots, Method B; the seeds in whole clusters, Method A or C, rubbed off the stems when dry.

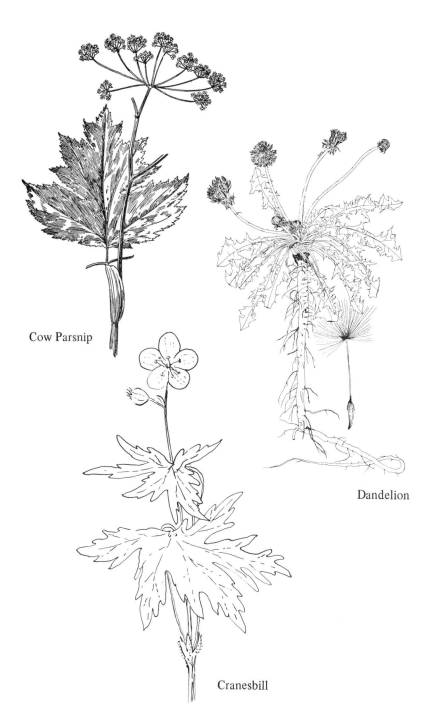

Cow Parsnip

Dandelion

Cranesbill

MEDICINAL USE: Cow Parsnip is a remedy for the stomach and nervous system. The root, which loses most of its acridity upon drying and should not be used fresh, is made into a tea (a teaspoon to a cup) and drunk for nausea that is of a persistent nature but does not progress to vomiting, as well as for acid indigestion or heartburn. In New Mexico it is often used for the gas and indigestion that accompanies a hiatus hernia, particularly in older women. The seeds are equally effective and if tinctured (fresh or dry), even a few drops on the tongue can settle the most unsettled stomach. Although not as antiseptic as oil of cloves, the seed tincture is a good temporary analgesic when applied to a sore tooth and is far less irritating to the gums. The root or seeds act as an antispasmodic to the intestinal tract and will help quiet tenesmus or cramping of the large intestine and the lower (ileum) section of the small intestine. It can sooth a spastic colon caused by mucous membrane inflammations but is less effective when it is of a distinctly nervous origin. It may help bronchial spasms and will both increase menstrual flow and relax uterine cramps. Like its relatives Angelica and Oshá, Cow Parsnip contains sufficient sterols and saponins to make it inadvisable to use it during a delicate pregnancy. In New Mexico a strong tea is made from the dry or wilted roots and poured into the bath water of a recently paralyzed person. This is repeated once a day until some nerve function has returned or the therapy has brought no apparent relief. Also, in northern New Mexico, a poultice or strong tea is applied to the face for tic douloureux (trigeminal neuralgia) particularly where there is some motor paralysis, and for *aigre;* a temporary paralysis of the face, neck, or arms that is attributed to bad night air or drafts. The powdered root or seeds can be used as a poultice for sore muscles and joints, having a mild rubefacient effect.

CRANESBILL

Geranium caespitosum, G. richardsonii   Geraniaceae

OTHER NAMES: Wild Geranium, Spotted Geranium, "Alum Root," Geranium

APPEARANCE: These two species and several less frequent in our area are true geraniums, as opposed to the garden varieties which are plants of the genus *Pelargonium.* They are plants of the higher altitudes and the two most commonly encountered in the West. They have pretty five-petaled flowers with ten stamens and palmate leaves, the apex of the lobes usually further notched. The stems tend to be nodular where they branch and often take on a reddish tinge in summer, particularly in the middle forest. *G. caespitosum* is a many-branched perennial with numbers of violet flowers having parallel purplish veins, many basal leaves, and a fairly substantial single or branching root with a dark bark and pinkish pith. *G. richardsonii* has white or light pink flowers, also darker veined, but is a slighter plant with fewer stems and in crowded high meadow habitats sometimes only one. The first species has distinctly five-lobed leaves, the second often has only three. All true geraniums form seed bundles that resemble a thick needle or . . . a crane's bill. Geranium should not be picked before flowering since the immature plants are almost indistinguishable from young Larkspur or monkshood (aconite), both dangerous but with very dissimilar flowers.

HABITAT: The various members of this genera are found in abundance in all of our moist mountains; the coastal ranges and inland ranges of California, the Sierra Nevadas, and eastward through Arizona, Nevada, Idaho, Utah, Colorado, Wyoming, Montana, and New Mexico, in and above the Ponderosa belt.

COLLECTING: The roots at anytime after flowering, from early summer to late fall, Method B. To powder the dried root, crisp up slightly in a warm oven and run through a blender or grinder. The leaves, Method A, when just flowering in the early summer or late spring.

MEDICINAL USE: Cranesbill is an astringent, owing its effects to tannins and gallic acid. Like most astringents it needs direct contact with the inflamed or bleeding surface to be effective. The root or leaves in tea can be used as a gargle for a sore throat, mouth inflammations including thrush and monilia, tonsillitis, and the like. The root, a teaspoon boiled in a cup of water, is effective in catarrhal gastritis and will decrease vomiting caused by a stomach ulcer. The same tea can be used as an enema for bleeding piles, hemmorrhoids, and inflamed diverticula, a douche for vaginitis, and even a drink for its mild systemic astringency. This may bring about some relief for sick headaches, excess menstruation, or post partum bleeding. The crushed fresh plant or root powder made into a paste with water and applied to puss-filled ulcers or abrasions of the skin will remove the pyogenic membrane and allow draining and a reduction of pressure. The root, sliced when fresh, can be used as a first aid for gum or tooth infections, applied directly on the area in pain. A related species is used in Europe as a face wash to help eradicate acne when accompanied by oily skin on the cheeks and nose. The powdered root is useful for applying to shallow injuries of the skin as a hemostatic and first aid.

DANDELION

Taraxacum spp.   Compositeae

OTHER NAMES: Chicória, Consuelda, *Leontodon taraxacum*

APPEARANCE: This is such a common plant as to almost need no description. Several points should be made, however, since the name is sometimes applied loosely to other milky-sapped weeds with fluffy yellow flowers. Dandelion has no stems at all; all leaves and the hollow flower stems grow directly from the rootstalk. If the plant in question has any branched or divided stems, it is not Dandelion.

HABITAT: It may seem strange to include this ubiquitous weed in a book of mountain plants; however, it is so useful that many people pick the plant for herb use and, considering the monochromatic, almost seasonless nature of much weather in the West, plants found in such localities often lack much potency. The constituents of Dandelion vary at different times of the year and the distinct seasons of the mountains result in decidedly stronger roots and leaves. It may be found growing almost to timberline in all of our mountains.

COLLECTING: The leaves, Method C; the flowers, Method C; the roots, Method B. No part of the plant should be considered very potent after a year's storage.

MEDICINAL USE: The constituents of Dandelion are taraxasterol, taraxerol (both water insoluble), fructose, inulin, choline, pectin, and, in the early spring, mannite. The leaves also contain inositol. The effect of all this is that the leaves and the root are a safe diuretic, increasing both the water and waste products in the urine. If a fresh tincture is made of the early spring roots, frequent one-fourth-teaspoon doses may be used for kidney inflammations and for restorative therapy after hepatitis. All parts of the plant have a mild stimulating effect on the liver. A tablespoon of the root a day or a teaspoon of the fresh root tincture a day, consumed in small, frequent doses, will aid either liver or spleen congestion. There is virtually no toxic potential to Dandelion, and large quantities may be drunk. This is necessary in such traditional uses as dissolving urinary stones and gravel, where up to an ounce of the chopped root is boiled and drunk in several doses during a day, or two tablespoons of the tincture are drunk in water twice a day. This should be done for at least ten days. The root in tea will have little effect on constipation due to nervousness, diet, fevers, and such occasional causes, but acts reliably when it is chronic, related to age, long-term illness, or general intestinal blahs; a teaspoon of the root boiled in water three or four times a day. The ground roots can be lightly roasted in a frying pan or browned in the oven on a cookie sheet to make "Dandelion Coffee"; I personally find this a mild insult to both Dandelion and Coffee, but some people are quite fond of it. For medicinal uses it should still be boiled.

DODDER

Cuscuta spp.   Convolvulaceae

OTHER NAMES: Devil's Guts, Yerba sin Raíz (Herb Without Root)

APPEARANCE AND HABITAT: The only confusion in identifying Dodder could arise from not knowing it to be a plant. It has no leaves, no chlorophyll, and, at maturity, no roots. This relative of the morning glories does have flowers and seeds, however humble, and seedling Dodders sprout from fruit, form roots, and almost resemble a normal plant until a host is encountered. The long threadlike stems have suckerlike appendages which attach to a host, grow into the inner pith, and thereafter are parasitic on the host's juices, the root withering, flowers and seeds formed, and the whole cycle begun again. These threadlike stems may form large claustrophobic mats of waxy, glistening yellow orange "guts" that often stifle, dehydrate, and eventually kill the host. One might, from an automobile, think Dodder to be some exotic recording tape tossed from a thoughtless passing car. It is encountered periodically in all of the West, but is most common in the upper foothills and middle shrubby heights. Dodder will frequent nearly any plant in sight, but trees are resistant to its inroads, small plants die quickly, and it is most abundant on waist-high broad-leaved shrubs.

COLLECTING: Whole, dense mats, as devoid of the host plant parts as practical and dried by Method C or laid out on newspapers. The dried threads should be chopped into small pieces for tea.

MEDICINAL USE: A rounded teaspoon of the chopped plant is a good laxative-cathartic and smaller quantities, drunk every few hours, will aid in reducing spleen inflammations, lymph node swellings, and "liver torpor." It contains bergegin (cuscitin). Dodder is used by the Chinese for treating impotence.

DOGBANE

Apocynum androsaemifolium   Apocynaceae

OTHER NAMES: Black Hemp, "Indian Hemp," Hemp Dogbane, Lechuguilla

APPEARANCE: Dogbane is a tidy looking herb, forming one or several greenish brown stems, one to three feet in height. All parts of the plant are intensely milky when broken. The glabrous, completely smooth leaves grow in wide-spaced pairs on thin, strong, round stems, and are oval-lanceolate with small petioles that, like the main stems, turn reddish by summer. The leaves and the pink white terminal flower clusters have a distinctive drooping attitude. The seed pods are usually paired, forming long thin calipers that also hang downwards. The roots are smooth and straight, about the thickness of a large pencil, and creep underground so that plants two or three feet apart may spring from the same root. Dogbanes tend to cross-pollinate freely, and the three native species in the West end up in the midst of many botanical subspecies and varieties. This is the most common type. Another species, *A. cannabinum,* has rounder leaves without a downward slant and less showy greenish white flowers. In most of the West it is found in various atypical hybrid forms and frequently serves as another addition to the *Apocynum* genetic pool. *A. androsaemifolium* is usually found in the pure form.

HABITAT: Common throughout the mountains, from 3,500 to 9,000 feet. Although traditionally associated with waste places, in our states it is just as likely to grow in near-wilderness areas, frequenting clearings as well as trails and old roads.

COLLECTING: The creeping roots in the fall after the aboveground part has gone to seed—Method C.

MEDICINAL USES: With the exception of the feebler Milkweeds (*Asclepias*), Dogbane is the only recognized cardiac stimulant of the West. Traditionally, Dogbane is the name applied to *A. androsaemifolium* and Canadian Hemp to *A. cannabinum.* Dogbane is the more common and the safer for herb use. The two should not be interchanged indiscriminately, since the latter has distinctly different and more dangerous effects on cardiac function and, considering the various varieties and probable variations in strength, is not appropriate for herbal or crude drug use. Both plants have similarities in pharmacology and use to *Stropanthus,* a drug plant used like digitalis and preferred to it in European medical practice. Dogbane must be used with caution, since it has definite toxic potential, but it is safe in doses of a "00" capsule or less. The active substances in Dogbane are apocynin, apocynamarin (stropanthidin), and traces of cymarin, androsin, and several sterols. Small doses of this witches' brew act as a vasoconstrictor, slowing and strengthening the heartbeat and raising the blood pressure. It is a strong diuretic, useful in cardiac dropsy and the like, but authorities differ as to whether it increases urine by irritation of the kidneys or dilation of the renal artery, or both. In fact, one of the reasons preventing its more frequent use in medicine is the variability of absorption, metabolization, effects, and pharmacology. A safe and reliable dose is a single "0" capsule of the powdered root a day, this acting as a mild cardiac tonic, diuretic, and antirheumatic. A gram or more will cause vomiting and several grams act as a strong irritant to the mucous and serous membranes. It has been used with success by homeopaths for alcoholism; a total of one-fourth to one-half teaspoon of the powdered root is drunk in tea during the course of a day in small, frequent doses. This is supposed to aid in the withdrawal symptoms but should not be continued for more than a week or so. The powdered root will also promote perspiration when applied locally and is a valuable counter-irritant .

Two common books on herbs contain serious errors about Dogbane. In *Back to Eden* by Jethro Kloss, the author makes reference to "Indian Hemp" but applies the Latin name of Jaborandi to what is presumably either Dogbane or Canadian Hemp, since the uses listed are the traditional Eclectic therapies that employ the latter plants. Jaborandi, however, is not related to the Apocynaceae and is in fact a well-known crude drug, the source of pilocarpine. Since Jaborandi leaves are widely available through herb stores for use as a hair rinse, a confusion arising from this book could be disastrous; two of the illnesses for which he recommends

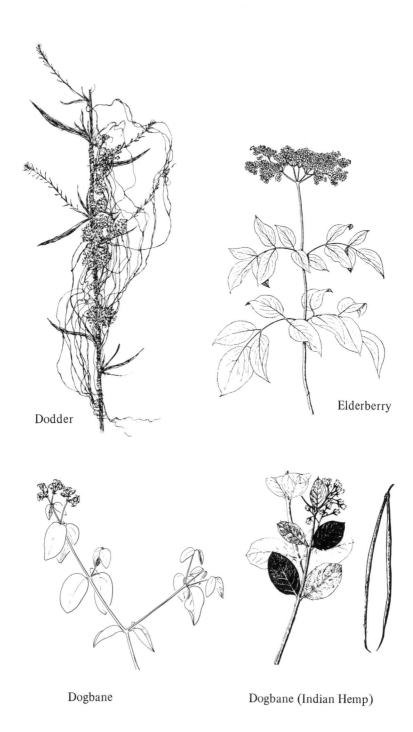

Dodder

Elderberry

Dogbane

Dogbane (Indian Hemp)

"Indian Hemp" are asthma and pleurisy, conditions that Jaborandi, i.e., pilocarpine, can severely aggravate. In *Indian Herbology of North America* by Alma Hutchins, a peculiar book at best, the author confuses Dogbane with *Cannabis sativa* and lists therapies for these two wildly dissimilar plants as if they are identical. The only similarities shared by hemp (marijuana) and Dogbane and Canadian Hemp are the long, tough stem fibers in the three plants that have been variously used for rope manufacturing.

OTHER USES: Dogbane, because of its counterirritating effects, can stimulate hair growth through its vasodilation and mild irritation of the follicles—a teaspoon of the root is boiled in a cup of water and the tea applied to the hair as a final rinse.

ELDERBERRY
Sambucus spp.   Caprifoliaceae

OTHER NAMES: Elder, Red Elder, Flor Sauco

APPEARANCE: Varies from a many-branched shrub to a small tree. The leaves are compound, with two to four pairs of leaflets and a single leaf at the tip. Elder can be confused with ash, the latter frequently found with similar compound leaves; some ashes have alternate leaves while those of Elder, even including branches, are always paired. Further, the seeds of the ash are winged while Elder grows bright red or purple berries. Elder blooms in late spring through to summer, and the flowers occur in dense, flat, or slightly pyramidal clusters, forming delicate cream-colored masses with a pleasant, slightly rancid scent. Berries can be bright red, frosted blue, or purple, with the same shape of cluster as the flowers.

HABITAT: From lower coastal ranges in California to fairly moist hillsides and foothills of Arizona and southern New Mexico. Stemmy red-berried shrubs can be found from 7,500 feet to 10,000 feet in northern Arizona and New Mexico, and north to Canada.

COLLECTING: Red Elderberries can be rather toxic; blue berries are preferable. Pick whole clusters of flowers or berries, not individual ones; they dry more reliably and can be removed from the stems when dry (Method C). The leaves and bark of many species can mildew and turn black if they are bundled. This is avoided by drying whole branches singly and removing the leaves and bark afterwards.

MEDICINAL USE: The most frequent use of Elder is to stimulate sweating in dry fevers. The flowers are the mildest and safest form of the plant, even suitable to be given to small children with equal parts of peppermint as a weak tea—a home remedy of ancient usage for breaking fevers. Caution should be used for those occasional children with histories of high fevers and convulsions; once in awhile the tea can raise the temperature slightly along with its stimulation to perspiration. Otherwise, the combination is quite safe. The leaves have the same use, although stronger and more energetic; suitable for adults. They also have a mild laxative effect. The flowers and dried berries are useful as a diuretic and have been used for centuries as an aid to rheumatism and arthritis, at least where a diuretic can be of aid in reducing symptoms. The bark, widely used in Europe, is not advisable in the West; our trees and bushes contain larger amounts of both hydrocyanic acid and sambucine, a nauseating alkaloid found mostly in the bark and root as well as the fresh plant. In fact it is advisable when making Elderberry jam or wine to strain out the seeds, as they contain both substances.

OTHER USES: As mentioned, the berries make an excellent and delicious jam and a potent, if slightly peculiar wine. Only the blue and purple berries are used—the red-berried species can be mildly toxic. Those berries facing east and west where the sun has shone directly have a sweeter taste and less bitterness. The fresh flowers steeped in water overnight or the commercially available Elder Flower Water is a widely used face conditioner. The skin of the face and neck is daubed with the liquid every evening, to tone the skin and allegedly to lighten freckles.

CULTIVATION: Best from nursery stock.

ESCOBA de la VIBORA
Gutierrezia spp.   Compositeae

OTHER NAMES: Matchweed, Snakebroom, Broomweed, Yerba de la Víbora, Collálle

APPEARANCE: A small, many-stemmed upright shrub with numerous narrow leaves and many little yellow flower clusters, three to eight blooms in a bunch, with small, scaly overlapping bracts. The plant has a resinous or waxy finish and when crushed gives off a slight piney scent. Perennial, new growth and previous dead stems are intermixed in the same bush. An insignificant bush, reaching an insignificant height, with insignificant leaves and flowers, its appearance is so common and uninteresting as to approach . . . insignificance.

HABITAT: High, dry slopes, mesas, flats, and the like, it is found in almost any area from the eastern two-thirds of California north and eastwards where there is enough moisture to support an undergrowth but not enough to support main forests, from above the creosote (*Larrea*) belt to and above the Piñon/Juniper belts, from 5,000 to 9,500 feet.

COLLECTING: Method A.

MEDICINAL USE: A cup of the finely chopped herb is steeped for thirty minutes in a quart of water, strained, and the tea added to a hot bath to alleviate the pain of arthritis and rheumatism. Like other palliative treatments, it won't cure anything, but it is effective in reducing inflammation and pain and, unlike many other herb baths for these conditions, such as chaparral (hediondilla), Tobacco, Jimson Weed, or marijuana, it can be repeated as often as necessary. A respected, almost revered *remedio* among Hispanic New Mexican and Arizona peoples, where a tea of the herb is usually drunk while bathing in it. The tea may also be drunk for stomach ache, especially in the morning, and as a treatment for excessive menstruation. Although by no means a heroic medicine, it is common, safe, and may sometimes work so well for joint inflammations as to supplant salicylate (aspirin) treatments.

EVENING PRIMROSE   (see color plate)
Oenothera hookeri, O. biennis   Onagraceae

OTHER NAMES: Tree Primrose, Flor de Santa Rita

APPEARANCE: These species and several less common are basically biennials, forming long-leaved rosettes the first year that are distinctive for the pronounced light green vein running the length of each leaf. In most areas the plant blooms the second year and dies that fall. The flowering plant, which is the form used, attains a height of two to five feet, the leaves and unbranched stem finely haired. The leaves are lance-shaped and possess a pronounced center vein, light in color like the first-year leaves. The single stem, coarse and tough, only branches slightly in wet years, enough to accommodate a flower or two. The root is turniplike and slightly peppery when raw. The striking flowers are bright yellow and slightly luminescent at night, blooming through summer and fall. In early summer the flowers only open in the late afternoon, hence their name. They grow at or near the top of the stem, from one to several blooming simultaneously, and turn salmon or orange when faded. The seed pods are little ridged cylinders an inch in length, crowded around the stem below the flowers. In long growing seasons the stem may accommodate two feet of seed pods and still be blooming at the top. By late summer the flowers will be blooming all day. There are many varied smaller Evening Primroses with either white, yellow, or pink flowers, all becoming reddish upon fading, but only the upright varieties are used.

HABITAT: From sea level to 9,000 feet, but most common in the mountains where they grow along streams, old fallow fields, roadsides, and in various wet places. Established in nearly all watersheds.

COLLECTING: Flowering tops Method A or Method C, depending on the length of stems; early summer preferable because of the fewer seed pods. Roots are split and dried as in Method B.

MEDICINAL USE: The root, fresh or dried, is chopped and boiled slowly in twice its volume of honey to make a cough syrup both soothing and somewhat antispasmodic. A tablespoon every three or four hours as needed. The tops can be used similarly. The herb possesses diuretic function and both root and herb have a sedative effect on some individuals. It has some laxative effect and can suppress both skeletal and smooth muscle pain, particularly in the reproductive organs. Evening Primrose is variable in its effects, both because of locality and species and because of personal sensitivities, but it can be a prime remedy for some individuals. As common as the plant is, it should be tried. Some of its effects can be attributed to the physiologically active amounts of potassium nitrate present in all parts of the plant. It also functions to some degree as a stimulant to the vagus nerve. Recommended dose: one to three teaspoons a day of the root or leaves in tea.

OTHER USES: The leaves are serviceable as cooked greens (although not exceptional) and the root is a good boiled vegetable, particularly in first-year plants. In foraging terms, this makes Evening Primrose one of the few widespread wild root vegetables in the West. Like most wild veggies, however, a somewhat acquired taste.

CULTIVATION: Seeds sown at random in October in moist ground.

FALSE SOLOMON SEAL

Smilacina racemosa   Liliaceae

OTHER NAMES: Solomon's Plume, *Vagnera racemosa, Convallaria racemosa*

APPEARANCE AND HABITAT: This is an attractive, striking plant of deep forests and rich soil, found above the Ponderosa belt in all the higher moist mountains of the West, from 7,000 to 10,000 feet. The unbranched stems usually form colonies and range from two to three feet in length, gracefully arched, rarely upright. The individual leaves are bright green and parallel veined, fairly large with a roundly pointed shape and a stem-clasping habit. The main stems tend to zigzag slightly

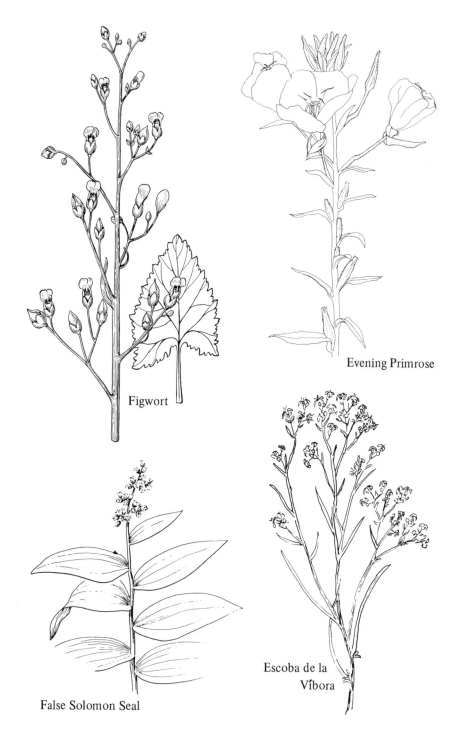

Figwort

Evening Primrose

False Solomon Seal

Escoba de la
Víbora

from leaf to leaf, and terminate in small alternate clusters of creamy white flowers that ripen into dark-spotted red berries. The rootstalk is horizontal and creeping, covered with round scars and nodules, with several leafing stems growing from various points along its fleshy length.

COLLECTING: The roots dug at any time, dried intact, Method C, and chopped finely for storage.

MEDICINAL USE: The root is an effective demulcent and expectorant for the inflammatory stages of lung infections and sore throats and will also facilitate the softening and upward movement of mucus in the bronchials. The root tea is also of value in frontal headaches caused or accompanied by indigestion. The tea is made by boiling a scant to rounded teaspoon in a cup of water for at least fifteen minutes, to be drunk at body temperature. The root and flowers have a feeble digitalis-like effect due to the presence of several of the *Convallaria* glycosides in minute quantities, but would probably have little therapeutic value. False Solomon Seal does have an occasional history of use in folk medicine for heart problems and may have some very mild effect, but this usage more than likely was brought about because of its close resemblance and botanical relation to *Convallaria* (lily of the valley), a former cardiac stimulant not found in our area. A smaller relative, *S. stellata,* is a slighter plant with almost identical appearance found in the same general areas as False Solomon Seal or growing directly with it. Although the roots are much smaller, *S. stellata* may be used in the same manner.

FIGWORT (see color plate)
Scrophularia spp.   Scrophulariaceae

OTHER NAMES: Scrofula Plant, Carpenter's Square

APPEARANCE: Figwort is a tall, slightly weedy plant, ranging from three feet, slender, and spreading in the California species, *S. californica,* to as tall as six feet and robust in the Arizona and New Mexican mountains. This latter variety, *S. lanceolata,* has also been called *S. nodosa* and *S. marylandica* in manuals, and is the predominant species outside of California, with upright, thick stems that are four sided in younger plants and eight sided in older ones. The leaves are large and oval-triangular, serrated, and often have secondary leaves growing from the axils of the main opposite leaves. The California plant, also found periodically in Arizona and Nevada, has smaller, more triangular leaves and it branches more readily; it, too, has a square stem with opposite leaves. The overall visage is like Catnip or Nettles, except that most varieties are smooth and hairless. The main stems in both varieties may turn reddish in the fall, and plants in the California coastal ranges have a dark maroon green tinge. Figwort flowers have a peculiarly immature look about them, forming little clusters of paired semiopened blossoms spaced along the terminal spikes. They are little fat cylinders with five lobes at the mouth, the upper two larger than the lower three. Colors vary from brown maroon to rust-tinged green, maturing into capsules filled with little dark wrinkled seeds.

HABITAT: The California Figwort grows in abundance in the coastal ranges, inland mountains through Mt. Pinos, and the Tehachapi and Sierra Nevada ranges, up to 6,500 feet. A downy variety is native to the higher altitudes of the Panamint and White Mountains, through to Nevada. In Arizona the species intergrade, and the typical *S. lanceolata* grows from the Gila and Sierra Blanca ranges of New Mexico, north to Wyoming, usually above 8,000 feet. *S. coccinea* of the southern mountains between Arizona and New Mexico is an endangered species and must not be picked; the other varieties are widespread, however.

COLLECTING: The aboveground plant in early or middle summer, Method A. For a fresh tincture or ointment, use the whole plant, finely chopped; for tea, remove the often thick major stems after drying, retaining the smaller stems, leaves and flowering tops, and seeds.

MEDICINAL USE: The old Doctrine of Signatures held the plant useful for skin eruptions because of the glandular nodes found on the roots and leaves of the main European species. This happens to be the case, which does not reflect the validity of that old tradition, so much as the ability of old physicians to find something in the plant's appearance to relate to its previous empirical use. Figwort could just as easily, by that doctrine, have been used for the following: mouth problems (the shape of the flowers), heart disease (the shape of some leaves), cuts and abrasions (leaf serrations), or ligament problems (the form of the stems), not to mention clotting blood (the color of the flowers). Since it did obviously have use in skin conditions, based on long folk use, it wasn't too hard to attribute this to the root nodules—after the fact, as it were. So did, and does, Homo sapiens fit the facts to the theory, the theory arising from a need to make a chaotic universe fit neatly into horse stalls.

The fresh tincture or a strong tea can be applied to fungal infections of the skin, ranging from cradle cap to athlete's foot, and can further help eczema, rashes, burns, or hemorrhoids. The dried plant may be drunk in a tea (a scant tablespoon or less of the tops in a cup of water) for hives, back and chest eruptions, and as a general blood purifier/alterative. It also has a mild sedative effect. The fresh tincture makes a good wash for most skin disorders, and a salve may be made by mashing or blending the fresh plant with an equal volume of vegetable oil. The mash should be allowed to stand for at least two weeks, strained or expressed through a cloth, and sufficient beeswax added to the slightly warmed oil to form an ointment consistency on cooling. It should be stirred once or twice while cooling to disperse the water and oil solubles. The active constituents are a stereoptene, propionic acid, and acetic acid.

FREMONTIA

Fremontia californica   Sterculiaceae

OTHER NAMES: Flannel Bush, California Slippery Elm, *Fremontodendron californica*

APPEARANCE AND HABITAT: A tall, rather handsome plant, with bluntly palmate, thickly fuzzy leaves and large orange to yellow showy single flowers. These have five "petals," actually calyxes masking as petals. Fremontia has the general appearance of a stubby, fuzzy hibiscus. This hearty shrub or treelet grows in canyons and rocky granite hillsides in most of the western half of mountainous southern California, and reappears in isolation in central Arizona. In both localities it will be found between the altitudes of 3,500 and 6,000 feet. The bush blooms in late spring and early summer, often dropping most or all of its leaves in late summer or during severe droughts.

COLLECTING: The leafy branches, Method A, the bark, Method D, or simply stuffed loosely in a shopping bag until dry. The dried bark should be chopped into small pieces and ground or run through a blender to reduce it to a usable coarse, fibrous powder. Its emollient properties will remain indefinitely. Plants in Arizona are infrequent, so pick sparingly, and only from substantial stands.

MEDICINAL USE: The leaves and especially the bark serve the same functions as slippery elm bark *(Ulmus fulva)* of commerce; Fremontia is one of the best possible teas for sore throats and irritated, ulcerous stomachs. A large pot of tea (two tablespoons to a pint of water), drunk within an hour, will bring up obstinate, dry mucus from the bronchials. The chopped bark is also used as a drawing poultice or as a base for counterirritants.

CULTIVATION: The seeds, planted in the fall, preferably on a well drained slope. Water freely in the spring, sparingly during the summer, if to be used for medicine, more often if ornamental.

GENTIAN (see color plate)

Gentiana spp.   Gentianaceae

OTHER NAMES: Blue Gentian, Purple Gentian, Fringed Gentian, Gentiana, Gall Plant

APPEARANCE: Particularly in their high subalpine habitat, Gentians are a visually distinctive group of plants. The whole plant tends to be smooth and waxy and seldom more than a foot in height. The leaves are opposite, bright green, and stem clasping, sometimes little more than overlapping scales. The annual species often form only single stems, the perennials several to many, the latter with distinct rootstalks or tubers, the former with thin, threadlike roots. By far the most common flower color is purple blue, and the shapes are funnelform, tubular, or bell-like, with parallel veins and, in some species, many parallel crepey involutions. In some varieties only the floral tips are colored, whereas in other types the whole flower and calyx are blue purple. There may be a single terminal flower or many blossoms growing out of the leaf axils in a steplike formation. The Fringed Gentians have flowers with many deep notches in the corolla. There are a few Gentians in the eastern part of our range, usually at or above timberline, with light yellow flowers and a few tiny blue flecks. The chemical Gentian Violet has no connection with the plant other than its . . . and their . . . distinctive color.

HABITAT: Go to the nearest mountains above 8,000 feet, and you will find Gentians in the wet meadows and bogs. If it is middle or late summer they are easily identified by their bright flowers. The higher you go, the more plants there will be, reaching a maximum distribution between 9,500 and 10,500 feet, except for the San Bernardino and San Jacinto ranges where the optimum level is 8,000 feet.

COLLECTING: In the perennial varieties, collect the root and dry loosely; the annuals are picked, rootlet and all, Method A.

MEDICINAL USE: The constituents of the Gentians always vary somewhat, but nearly all contain the bitter glycoside gentiopicrin, several bitter amorphic substances, gentisic acid, several sugars peculiar to the genera, and, in the perennial roots, several water insoluble sterols. Gentiopicrin (for malaria) and gentisic acid (for rheumatic inflammations) are still used in pharmacy. The Gentians are, above all, perhaps the best stomach tonics in the plant kingdom, and certainly the most specific in the West. The best possible remedy for the person with chronic indigestion and dyspepsia in the evening. The root or chopped herb is steeped, a scant teaspoon in a cup, until it reaches body temperature, and drunk one-half hour before meals, particularly the evening meal. It is an excellent tonic for the aged or bedridden, especially when there is little appetite and food causes a gagging, boluslike sensation in the stomach, with the stomach still unemptied many hours later. A good remedy for those with excess stomach acid but equally useful when there is insufficient hydrochloric acid secretion.

The fresh plant in tincture is the optimum form of ingestion and can be used in great dilution, a few drops in some warm water. The plant is intensely bitter and is definitely an acquired or tolerated taste, but it has none of the aftertaste of other bitter herbs, and there is a certain pristine nastiness about the tea that makes it in some peculiar way an almost welcome beverage when it is needed. For those with chronic stomach and intestinal problems the following tincture compound can be a godsend. By volume, mix ten parts of the fresh plant or root with five parts of orange peel, one part ground cardamom seed, five parts honey, and twice their total volume in brandy. Steep for a week, strain or express through a cloth, and bottle for use. The tea or tincture of Gentian alone can be found useful for fevers and joint inflammations that are aggravated in the evenings. Excess amounts of Gentian may cause nausea and stomach disturbances, but considering its bitterness, only the most grimly resolute self-punishing person could manage such a quantity.

CULTIVATION: It is difficult to bring Gentian down from the mountains to a garden, but dormant roots or tubers (late fall, early spring) from perennial plants may take in an acidic, mulchy, wet but well drained area.

GRINDELIA

Grindelia spp.   Compositeae

OTHER NAMES: Yerba del Buey, Gumweed, Rosinweed, Tarweed

APPEARANCE: The leaves are green to blue green, somewhat spade shaped, and clasp the stem without a leafstalk. They are slightly toothed. When it is in bloom the plant is about three feet in height and the many sticky yellow flowers are surrounded by pincushionlike bracts. The young flowers and buds are covered in a thick, milky exudate that smells balsamic, a device that insures pollination if insects fail, and which gives rise to its name of Gumweed, for it can be chewed like chicle.

HABITAT: Found in open gravelly areas, around buildings and vacant lots, in disturbed earth, and along roadsides at elevations from 3,000 to 8,000 feet. From coastal ranges in California to the plains states, in southern Arizona and New Mexico mountains, northwards to Wyoming.

COLLECTING: The buds and flower heads when first in bloom, the leaves before flowering. Flowers, Method C; leaves, Method A.

MEDICINAL USES: An official drug plant in European medicine, it has been deleted recently in the United States. As a tea the leaves and flowers can be used interchangeably. For tincturing the flowers are preferable. As a tea for bronchitis and wherever an expectorant is needed. It is a useful antispasmodic for dry hacking coughs, alone or combined with Yerba Santa, a tablespoon in tea as needed. The tincture is especially useful for bladder and urethra infections, one-fourth teaspoon in water every four hours. Topical use of the tincture or a poultice of the crushed flowers is often helpful in poison oak inflammations. A mild sedative and cardiac relaxant, although not always reliable. Its unpleasant bitterness makes it useful as a mild stomach tonic.

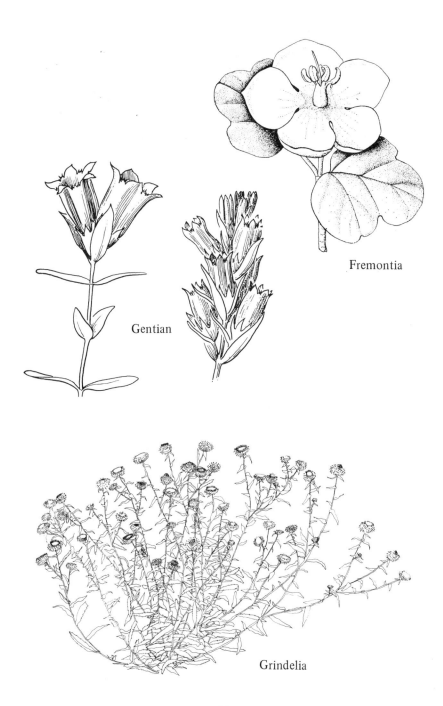

Fremontia

Gentian

Grindelia

OTHER USES: The young leaves make a pleasantly aromatic, slightly bitter tea, and the young gummy flowers can be used as chewing gum. The leafless stems can be bound together to make brooms.

CULTIVATION: A rather undecorative plant at best, about the only possible reason for purposely growing this tacky weed would be for medicinal use. If you do so, throw the seeds out into the worst soil you can find and then disavow them when they sprout.

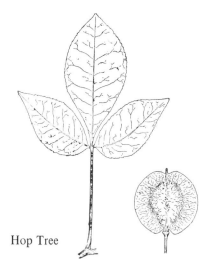

Hop Tree

HOP TREE

Ptelea trifoliata, etc.   Rutaceae

OTHER NAMES: Wafer Ash, Swamp Dogwood

APPEARANCE: A large shrub or small tree seldom growing above ten feet in height, usually five or six feet. The leaves are in threes, pointed-oval, the side leaflets without stem, the center having a petiole. Hop Tree rarely has "green green" leaves; off-colors of dusty green, blue green, or olive drab are customary. The undersides of the leaflets are lighter than the tops. The branch bark is usually reddish brown but may be olive or brown green in moister areas, only turning darker in the fall. The distinctive fruit is egg-shaped and flat, forming dense clusters of little wafers that resemble the samaras of the ash tree and offhandedly resemble rolled oats with a thick center. The entire plant, like most members of the Rutaceae, has a slightly disagreeable odor.

HABITAT: Hop Tree is a common plant in the medium altitudes of Arizona, Nevada, New Mexico, Utah, and Colorado, but does not make it to southern California, not getting much further south than the Bay Area. Southern California, in fact, is one of the few areas in the country where Hop Tree does not grow. The botanical nomenclature is rather fuzzy, with the widely varying shapes of leaf and fruit making species differentiation difficult. Many botanists would like to lump the whole mess into *P. trifoliata,* whereas others might see a doctoral dissertation in a further redundant division into species, subspecies, and variety. It is most frequently found in the upper Juniper/Piñon, lower Ponderosa belts, in dry gullies, mesas, and exposed areas, from 4,000 to 8,000 feet.

COLLECTING: The root bark or tree bark in autumn, the leaves and fruit in late summer, Methods D, C, and A respectively.

MEDICINAL USE: The active constituents are the peculiar volatile oil of the plant, the alkaloid berberine, and the amino acid arginine, the latter two with stimulating effects on the liver. The leaves and fruit are effective bitter tonics, a scant teaspoon steeped in water and drunk shortly before meals when chronic poor digestion is being treated or after a particularly greasy meal resulting in heartburn or dyspepsia. An example of a Hop Tree Need would be a medium pepperoni pizza at 8:00 p.m., a pitcher of beer at 8:30–9:00 p.m., two glasses of Chianti at 10:30 p.m., dancing and peanuts until 12:30 p.m., . . . until 2:00 a.m., retiring (after a shared cigarette) at 2:15 a.m., and an esophagus acid bath at 3:22 a.m. At such a time the plant-wise lady or gentleman would curse, stumble into the kitchen, and fix a cup of Hop Tree tea. The leaves have been used for treatment of roundworms and pinworms, one to two tablespoons in tea during a day until symptoms subside. This is probably inadvisable for children, since the volatile oil can cause nausea in some young people. The bark is a specific for fevers accompanying intestinal malfunctions, gout, and rheumatism, a scant teaspoon of the chopped bark boiled for fifteen minutes in a covered vessel and drunk as needed. This is most appropriate in the evenings.

OTHER USES: The fruit has long been used in place of Hops in the brewing of beer; hence its name Hop Tree.

CULTIVATION: From the seeds collected in the fall. It prefers slightly alkaline soil.

HOPS

Humulus americanus   Moraceae

OTHER NAMES: Zarsa, Lupulo, *Humulus neomexicana*

APPEARANCE: Hops bears a superficial resemblance to the Grape plant, having large, opposite, three-(usual) to seven-lobed leaves with a coarse, hairy surface. The stems of this vine twist from left to right around any handy bush or tree, sometimes climbing forty feet or more up Poplars or Willows, other times forming dense trailing mats down moist slopes. Single stems can exceed thirty feet in length with several stems intertwined in braidlike formations. The flowers are inconspicuous, dioecious, and eventually mature into the "hops," the plump oval cylinders formed by overlapping membranous scales. These are very light, one to one and one-half inches long, with a light yellowish green to amber (ripe) color and a slightly garliclike scent. These fruit (technically called strobiles) form open clusters on the ends and undersides of the stems. The stems are generally green, although thin brownish bark is sometimes formed on the oldest parts of larger plants.

HABITAT: Our native species is found in Utah, Arizona, and the Rockies from New Mexico northwards. It does not reach westward to California but escaped plants of the European species *(Humulus lupulus),* cultivated for beer, are seen on occasion in northern California. The native species is found from 5,500 feet to over 9,000 feet, in very moist forest, shady embankments, the lips of forest meadows, and along streams. It is widespread but not particularly common in our area, becoming profuse in the central Rockies.

COLLECTING: The strobiles should be picked in early fall as they have reached full size and lost their greenish color. Care should be taken to begin drying as soon after picking as possible since they darken and mildew easily. If they form dense clusters it is advisable to clip the whole section, stem and all, removing the fruit when ready to dry. If Method C is used, do not layer strobiles more than three inches thick and turn frequently. It is better to dry with very low heat (125–150 degrees) in the oven with the door slightly ajar on a wire screen or burlap bag. If they're deteriorating rapidly, it is best to tincture.

MEDICINAL USE: Hops has four basic effects on the body. It is a sedative, bitter tonic, anodyne, and antibiotic. Hops is perhaps the ideal remedy for a nervous stomach, its aromatic bitterness acting to stimulate and redefine stomach functions, its sedative effects relaxing the individual and slightly dampening the related dominance of the sympathetic nervous system. The dose is three to five strobiles in hot water or a scant or rounded tablespoon of the chopped dried plant, drunk at body temperature. Oddly enough, several clinical tests "disproved" the sedative qualities of Hops and found they had no physiological activity on the nervous system, and yet anyone who drinks much of the tea will tend to fall asleep or get groggy. Hops are a safe sedative for children, relaxing muscle tension, spasms, and the general irritability associated with colds and such. Use one-half to one teaspoon in one-half cup of water for tea. Hops have helped colonic spasms, nervous dysentery, and intestinal cramps in general, particularly in people who eat quickly or have coffee and doughnuts for breakfast and a bologna sandwich for lunch.

A strong tea of the plant can help relieve toothaches and minor body pains, from rheumatism to sciatica, particularly when the pains are interfering with sleep. A sure cure for insomnia brought on by trashing out on oyster stew or candied watermelon peels (and similar gastric manias) shortly before retiring. When the usual nightmares concerning Attila the Hun or the Teapot Dome Scandal ensue and the indulger is unable to reconcile several realities (including being awake with a stomach ache at three in the morning), the Hops can be brewed up. For maximum benefit, the newly dried strobiles can be tinctured and one-half to one teaspoon of it used in warm water in place of the tea. When tinctured the potency remains indefinitely, whereas the herb is not of much use past six or eight months. Hops contains at least two antibiotic substances, humulon and lupulon, neither particularly water soluble, but both effective on staph and other skin bacteria. This is the reason that Hops is used in the making of beer, since they retard spoilage and preserve. Both substances being alcohol soluble, the tincture is an excellent treatment for skin sores, abcesses, and the like, applied every few hours until the inflammation is reduced, or the strobiles moistened with brandy or vodka, crushed, and applied as a hot poultice. Small pillows stuffed with Hops are a traditional remedy for insomnia (both Abraham Lincoln and George III slept on them), but the peculiar scent can get downright repulsive to some people, me included.

OTHER USES: The new shoots of May can be blanched by covering with cardboard or cloth for four or five days, cutting as far back on the stems as they are tender, and cooked like asparagus. The coarse leaves make a pleasant, slightly relaxing tea.

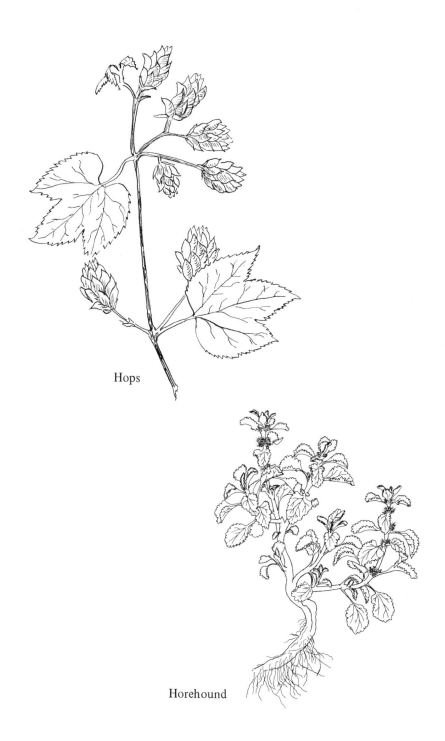

Hops

Horehound

HOREHOUND

Marrubium vulgare   Labiateae

OTHER NAMES: White Horehound, Mastranzo, Marrubio, Concha

APPEARANCE: The most distinguishing features are the white and wooly square stems, the downy oval and crenelated leaves, and the sagelike puffs of spiney flowers at the top of the stems. A distinctive, common, easily remembered member of the mint family. Unlike most of the family, Horehound has hardly any scent. The whole plant is strongly bitter. Plants in dry areas and full sun are hairier and appear lighter of hue; those in some shade and moisture tend to be darker with greener, less hairy stems. Dead flower twigs survive into the next year, leaving little barbed seed clusters to catch on the clothes and fur of bypassers. A perennial, many stemmed plant from one to two and one-half feet tall.

LOCATION: Throughout the United States in drier, sandy areas, vacant lots, and the like, particularly on abandoned land and old, disturbed earth. You are apt to find it anywhere that is not very pretty. It can be found at all altitudes.

COLLECTING: Method A, picked below the lowest pair of good leaves, right after full flower as the seed puffs start to get stiff.

MEDICINAL USE: An old and revered bitter expectorant. Pour a pint of boiling water over one-half ounce or handful of the chopped plant, steep for ten minutes, and drink during the day. It is bitter, so it can help to add several teaspoons of honey and a squeezed lemon or lime to the pint. It can be stored in the refrigerator during the day, one-half cup of the tea added to one-half cup hot water from the faucet for each cup. For coughs and lung congestion in general, a syrup is often preferable. This is my recipe (there are endless variations): Boil an ounce of Horehound in a pint of water for twenty minutes, strain, and reduce the liquid to a cup. Add two cups honey and stir over low heat. Remove from heat and add one ounce powdered slippery elm bark or powdered comfrey root, the juice from one lime, and one-half cup brandy. If you are fortunate enough to have some handy, several tablespoons of powdered Oshá Root can also be added. Mix thoroughly and bottle. Take a tablespoon or two as needed. The tea, drunk hot, will help reduce feverish coughs and promote sweating; drunk cold it is a good stomach bitter, stimulating both stomach and duodenal secretions. Chronic use for extended lengths of time can have hypertensive effects, however, particularly in relation to arterial tension.

OTHER USES: A substitute for Hops in beer, still sold as Horehound Ale in Europe.

CULTIVATION: Seeds sown in early spring in sandy, dry soil moistened for the occasion.

HORSETAIL

Equisetum spp.   Equisetaceae

OTHER NAMES: Scouring Rush, Shavegrass, Canutillo del Llano, Equisetum

APPEARANCE: During the Carboniferous age, the Horsetail family was the dominant group of plants in the world, reaching gigantic size; two basic Horsetails have survived to our day, mere miniaturizations. One is the hollow, jointed, and leafless Scouring Rush, the other the ferny Horsetail. This type, typified by *E. arvense,* has many crepey threadlike leaves cascading in whorls from the stem joints (see illustration, parts b and c), all parts covered in fine, lengthwise ridges and hollow except at the stem joints. The "horsetails" are actually sterile shoots; the fertile shoots grow in early spring, resembling small asparagus sprouts. The fertile stalks have a general pinkish green color, are very brittle, and die back before the main sterile growths. The sterile horsetails are the medicinal parts. The Scouring Rush, typified by *E. hyemele* (see illustration, part a), has no leaves, only degenerate scales around the joints of the stalks. It can be used like the Horsetail types, although it is somewhat less soluble as tea.

HABITAT: Stagnant water, bogs, sumps, slow-moving springs and creeks, shady banks, and the like. If not found directly in or near moisture, they are a reliable sign of a very high water table or former spring pools. They are found throughout the United States from sea level to 9,000 feet or higher.

COLLECTING: The green sterile shoots cut at ground level and bundled as in Method A. The Horsetail forms should be tied in small, loose bundles or they can mildew. Care should be taken not to collect along heavily fertilized ditches or meadows, as sufficient nitrates can be stored in the plant to render them somewhat toxic. Horsetail is also one of the plants that will collect selenium when it is present in the soil to any major degree.

MEDICINAL USES: An herb used in urinary tract disorders. In moderate doses a sure and safe diuretic, increasing both the volume of water and the acidity of the urine, which makes it useful for most lower urinary tract infections. Horsetail works best in small, frequent doses, a rounded teaspoon of the dried herb in tea three of four times a day until the inflammation has subsided. A source of silica (SiO_2) and aconitic acid ($C_6H_6O_6$), Horsetail will also aid in coagulation and help decrease bleeding. It is useful in excess menstruation, intestinal bleeding, and externally as a hemostatic. If large quantities are drunk at one time or if its use is continued for more than several weeks it can become an irritant to the urinary tract tissues and the intestinal mucosa. The alkaloid equisetin, which is found in differing quantities in the various species, is a substance that can act as a mild hypnotic but is somewhat toxic in large quantities of tea if it is present to any substantial degree.

OTHER USES: The leafless Scouring Rush, ridged with silica, can be bundled and dried, forming a scouring pad for cleaning and shining aluminum, copper, and wood. Equivalent to the finest grades of steel wool in polishing wood finishes, it was formerly a standard item with European cabinetmakers.

HOUND'S TONGUE

Cynoglossum officinalis   Boraginaceae

APPEARANCE: This naturalized European plant is usually a biennial and is often mistaken for either comfrey or Mullein. The long tapering leaves (up to seven inches in length) form a basal rosette the first year, with the leaves finely downy but not as hairy as Mullein or as coarse as comfrey. The second year the rosette grows upwards and forms long droopy scorpioid flower panicles, the funnelform blossoms densely packing the stems and varying on a single plant from rust red to lavender to purple colored. These mature into little burred seeds, flattened on one side and oval-triangular in shape. The root is light in color and carrotlike.

HABITAT: Common above 6,000 feet in New Mexico and Colorado, generally in shaded areas near farming or as high as 9,500 feet in mountain forests around camping and grazing. It is also found sporadically in the northern mountains of

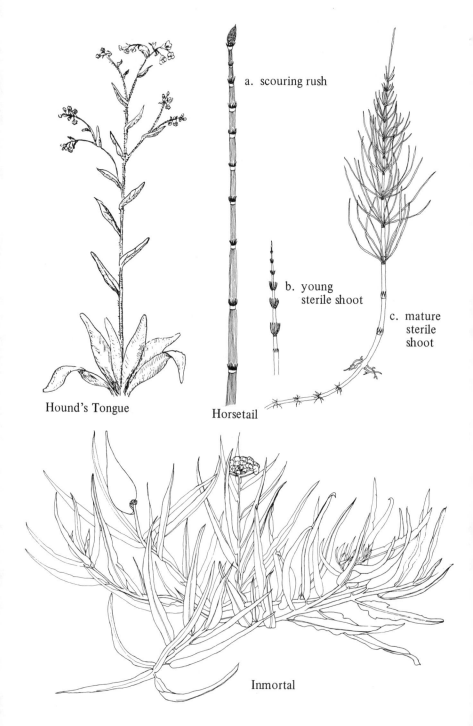

a. scouring rush

b. young
sterile shoot

c. mature
sterile
shoot

Hound's Tongue

Horsetail

Inmortal

Arizona (Flagstaff, Page) and Utah. I have encountered a few plants in the southern Sierra Nevadas and around Lake Arrowhead, but it is otherwise uncommon in southern California. Like so many other burr-seeded adventurers, it will come that way eventually.

COLLECTING: The herb and root in the summer, preferably when in full bloom. Method A or C.

MEDICINAL USE: Similar in use and effect to its close relative, comfrey, and like it, contains allantoin, the waxy purine metabolite so useful in treating skin and intestinal ulcerations. The root also contains an alkaloid, heliosupine. The plant makes an excellent tea for sore throat accompanied by a dry hot cough, a rounded teaspoon of the chopped root or tablespoon of the herb in water and sipped slowly. Like comfrey, the herb or root makes a good treatment for piles and hemorrhoids, drunk every evening.

INMORTAL (see color plate)

Asclepias asperula   Asclepiadaceae

OTHER NAMES: Antelope Horns, Spider Milkweed, *Asclepiodora decumbens, Asclepias capricornu*

APPEARANCE: Inmortal is a rather strange looking Milkweed. Seldom upright, it looks for all the world like a clump of coarse, trailing grass, at least until the big Milkweed pods begin to form in midsummer or the plant is bruised and the milky sap observed. The pods will sometimes grow outward in opposing pairs, a somewhat startling hornlike formation that gives rise to one of its common names, Antelope Horns. One of the most difficult of our medicinal plants to locate and identify, it is probably widespread. The seeds, however, are borne on the wind, across valleys and mountain ranges, making thick stands a rarity. The root is often gigantic for the comparatively small foliage, thick as a fist and with deeply furrowed brown gray bark in older plants, smooth barked with distinctive reddish tan longitudinal stripes along the side roots or in younger plants. The root is rather brittle, with a cream-colored milky-juicy pith. The roots creep tortuously under gravel, over rocks, and down slopes. Some plants can be shallow rooted, ending in little sweet-potato tubers. Most well established root systems disappear finally under three-ton boulders. The round flowers form inconspicuous little clusters around the upper stems.

HABITAT: Dry, rocky hillsides, both above and below the Juniper/Piñon belt, growing up into Ponderosa or down into Yucca flats. Difficult to typify because of its scattering seeding habits. Found sporadically in the Providence Mountains of California, foothills and dry mountains rimming the Mohave and Colorado deserts, Nevada, east through north and central Arizona and north and central New Mexico, to Nebraska and Arkansas . . . and who knows where else. Good hunting.

COLLECTING: The roots in the fall after seeding. The larger and older plants will frequently have the seeding stems of several years as dead stalks hanging below the new year's growth. Plants with several opened pod husks are generally worth digging; younger plants have one or two pods at the most. Any substantial portion of the root that is left in the ground will regrow the following year—hence its Spanish name, Inmortal. The ideal picking circumstance is a stand of several dozen plants growing up or down a moderate slope. Some of the roots will follow the slope downwards through loose gravel or dirt and can practically be lifted out with the fingers. Unfortunately, the majority will be so deeply embedded in large rocks and dense gravel that you will need a caterpillar tractor as the only appropriate digging tool and cut-and-fill as the only appropriate method. In dense soil, dig a hole around the root to a foot in depth, twist the upper part away, and forget the rest . . . it is seldom worth the labor involved. Dry loosely in a shallow box.

MEDICINAL USES: Outside the Spanish and Indian herbal tradition of New Mexico, Inmortal is virtually unknown. In its broad spectrum of effect and its level of function, however, it ranks as one of the dozen or so prime plant medicines found in the United States. It is a bronchial dilator and stimulates lymph drainage from the lungs; consequently, a medicine for asthma, pleurisy, bronchitis, and lung infections in general. One-half teaspoon of the dried root is boiled in water and drunk every three or four hours as long as necessary. The root is a mild but reliable cardiac tonic, particularly in congestive heart disorders, one-half teaspoon of the powdered root swallowed with water in the morning, either occasionally or for maintenance. Has no tendency to accumulate.

Inmortal is an effective menstrual stimulant, either for tardiness or for stimulating a scanty, painful period; one-half to one teaspoon in tea, once or twice. It has been used as an abortifacient up to the sixth week of pregnancy but is not reliable, and is more likely to cause nausea than a miscarriage. The tea drunk after childbirth or during labor will aid in shortening the uterine contractions afterward and decrease the time necessary for vaginal discharge or lochia. A small amount of the root taken several times during a day will stimulate the changeover from colostrum to milk production. Further, a small amount of the finely powdered root can be snuffed vigorously up each nostril to produce copious sneezing without irritation, which can clear up the most obstructed sinus. I am aware of no plant analysis to date, but the glycoside asclepiadin is undoubtedly present as well as, probably, a cardiac glycoside. Inmortal causes obvious vagus nerve stimulation. The root will stimulate perspiration at the onset of an infection and has a laxative effect.

CULTIVATION: Probably possible from the transplanted rootstock in the fall. The ripe, dark-centered seeds also could be used, probably without stratifying.

JIMSON WEED (see color plate)

Datura spp.   Solanaceae

OTHER NAMES: Thorn Apple, Datura, Stramonium, Toloache, Estramonio, Devil Weed, "Loco Weed"

APPEARANCE: Jimson Weed is a rank, smelly plant of large proportions with broad, dark green leaves and round, many-branching rubbery stems, all often blissfully insect ridden. The large trumpetlike flowers, uncurling like morning glories from the tubular calyx, are very light violet to purple with a delicious narcotic-sweet scent. They may run six inches in length and are large, showy, and spectacular. Compared to the rank foliage and large divided leaves, the blossoms seem to belong to another plant; often growing into six-foot malevolent clumps, Jimson Weed looks like a fugitive from a tropical rain forest. The seed pods are the size of golf balls and are covered with needle-sharp spines; despite the plant's toxicity and armaments, these pods are frequently worm ridden. If you are driving around in high desert foothills with nothing around you but gray dusty shrubs bearing little skimpy water-hoarding leaves and suddenly come across some plants

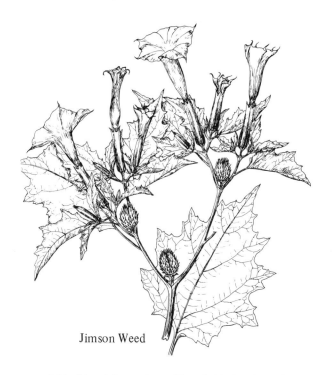

Jimson Weed

with large wasteful looking foliage, they will probably be either Jimson Weed or buffalo goard *(Curcubita foeditissima),* a many-branched ground vine with triangular sandpapery leaves. They both stink.

HABITAT: Large stands can be found in the driest, most desolate flats of the Mohave and Colorado deserts, but our several species of Jimson Weed generally inhabit foothills and drier mountains, from 2,500 to 7,000 feet. Single plants are uncommon; Jimson Weed generally forms stands in valleys, protected flats, and along dry washes. Isolated groups may follow along roads or irrigation ditches in the middle of nothing in particular. Unpredictable but common in distribution and probably found in every county of the West.

COLLECTING: The whole plant, uprooted if small, or several branches bundled together, Method A. For external use there is no advantage in collecting any one part of the plant unless it is to be used for smoking, in which case the leaves and flowers should be taken and rubbed fine after drying.

MEDICINAL USE: This is a plant that should never be taken internally for any reason. The primary alkaloid found in Jimson Weed is scopalamine, with varying smaller amounts of hyoscyamine and atropine, all highly toxic. The proportions found in different plant parts, species, and localities are extremely varied, making it highly unreliable even in trained hands for internal use. It is very useful for relaxing bronchial spasms in asthmatic attacks, the smoke from the leaves inhaled in any one of several ways. The "Asthma Powders" of older use were often only a mixture of equal parts of Jimson Weed and potassium nitrate (saltpeter), ground into a fine powder, ignited at the first sign of spasms, and inhaled. Simply sprinkling some of this dust on the flame of a cigarette lighter several times is often sufficient. The leaves may also be rolled into a cigarette with an equal amount of the leaves from any of the wild Sages *(Salvia* sp.). An older, tried and true mixture to smoke for asthma is equal parts (in weight) of Jimson Weed, Mullein leaves, and cubeb berries. The effect of inhaling a puff or two of Jimson Weed is a temporary numbing of bronchial enervation which relaxes the muscles; the smoke also acts to dry up the hypersecretions of the membranes. Why this method is no longer used is beyond my understanding. Frequent use decreases its effect, but the same is true of epinephrine and isoproterenol, the drugs used in asthma inhalers. Since the function of the Jimson Weed is almost completely local, there is no need to inhale enough to get into the bloodstream; the others all have strong systemic effects and can cause a rebound in some individuals, as well as a whole host of adverse reactions. For sinus inflammations a little smoke inhaled through the nostrils will bring some temporary relief to the swollen mucosa.

The fresh plant has the strongest potency and makes an excellent poultice or fomentation; when applied to painful joints or areas inflicted with neuralgia it acts as an analgesic and mild anti-inflammatory agent. Like Tobacco, a handful of the fresh or dried plant boiled in a large pot of water and the resultant tea added to a hot bath will relieve muscle pains and joint discomfort. Protracted use at one time can result in sufficient absorption of the alkaloids to cause drowsiness, however, and an elderly person or someone with restricted movement should not be left in overlong. Similarly, a cup of the chopped plant and a tablespoon of Cayenne Pepper, steeped in a quart of rubbing alcohol for at least a week, makes a good analgesic liniment. For hemorrhoids or piles, one part of the powdered plant is heated very slowly with lard, Vaseline, or lanolin (hydrous) for an hour, cooled, and applied as needed topically.

A final word of caution. The periodic attempts of some people to eat or smoke Jimson Weed to get high or hallucinate, based wrongly on good sources (the Castaneda books, as an example) or bad ones ("Herbal High" pamphlets or sleazy little ads in the back pages of drug culture periodicals . . . or sketchy rumor), can be very nasty indeed. The traditional uses of plants for euphoric, ritual, stimulant, or hallucinogenic purposes can be lumped into two categories. Those such as coffee, tobacco, marijuana, khaat, and even peyote can be, and usually are, part of socially accepted frivolities or rituals, consumed in that social milieu by average persons. Quite frankly, nearly every person on this planet takes something nearly every day to alter themselves, be it kola nuts, coca leaves, kava, betel nuts, tea, Coca Cola . . . even sugar. The other group of plants, however, are dangerous, toxic, and exact a strong physical price; to use them to a purpose takes experience and guidance until the desired reactions can be separated from the body toxicities and put to use. In traditional cultures where such ritual herbs are employed, they are used by ordained and trained holy men, shamans . . . specialists, if you will. Jimson Weed is one of these plants and should be left completely to those few men and women still trained in the traditions that call for this dangerous sacrament. To dabble in Jimson Weed for dilettante pseudoritual purposes or to try to get stoned with it is a silly, gratuitous, and dangerous thing. Things that make you feel good are legal, semilegal, or illegal but are widely known and generally available for the asking. The few relatively safe exotic plant drugs are rarely found outside the area of use and are even more rarely encountered in the contraband marketplace. Besides, Jimson Weed makes anyone feel absolutely wretched when taken internally.

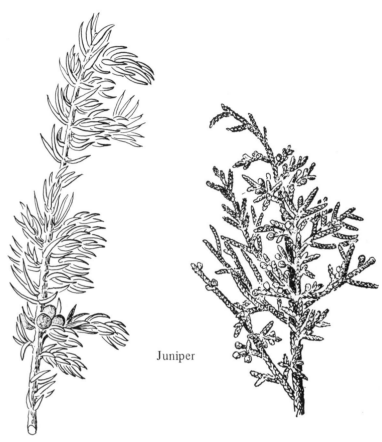

Juniper

Juniperus communis   *Juniperus monosperma*

JUNIPER   <small>(see color plate)</small>

Juniperus spp. Cypressaceae

OTHER NAMES: "Cedar," Cedron, Sabina

APPEARANCE: There are two general types of Junipers: small trees with dark olive green scaly, leafless twigs and the high altitude spreading shrub with sharp, pinelike needles. The seeds or fruit of the tree, like its leaves, are strongly aromatic, almost perfectly round, green initially, turning frosted blue by spring. The high altitude types are flattened shrubs, growing out in a rough circle until, in older plants, they may attain a circumference of ten or fifteen feet. The needle leaves are quite sharp and prickly with a bluish green color, somewhat lighter underneath. The large purple berries are green the first fall and are intermingled with mature berries from the previous year, generally clustered on the underside of the outer branches.

HABITAT: The tree Junipers are found at lower altitudes in dry foothills, from 1,500 feet in southern California to 8,000 feet in the Rockies. Sometimes forming pure stands, they are frequently found in an almost symbiotic relationship with the Piñon Pine, particularly in Arizona and New Mexico. The high altitude Junipers *(J. communus, J. sibirica,* and *J. montana)* are generally found above 8,000 feet to about 10,000 feet, with *J. sibirica* growing up to timberline.

COLLECTION: The berries when ripe (bluish or purple), the leaves whenever needed. Berries, Method C; leaves, Method A.

MEDICINAL USES: Primarily a urinary tract herb, most frequently used for cystitis and urethritis. The berries are the most effective. Use a teaspoon of crushed berries or a rounded teaspoon of the leaves, steeped in a covered cup of water for fifteen minutes and drunk, one to three cups a day. More effective and less irritating when combined with Uva Ursi, Manzanita, or Pipsissewa. Juniper should not be used when there is a kidney infection or chronic kidney weakness, as the oils are excreted in the urine and can be uselessly irritating to such inflammations. Munching a few berries an hour or so before meals will stimulate stomach secretions, i.e., hydrochloric acid and pepsin. The aromatic properties of all parts of Juniper plants have been used against bad magic, plague, and various negative influences in so many cultures, from the Letts to the Chinese to the Pueblo Indians, that there would seem to be some validity to considering the scent as beneficial in general to the human predicament. Overlapping traditions are useful in triangulating valid functions in folk medicine. If unrelated traditions say that Yarrow clots blood, it is easy to admit that such is probably the case; if they say that Juniper clears "bad vibes," many of us will back off and start to twitch skeptically. Our mechanistic approach to "primitivism" is too selective, accepting the possibility of drug effect on the one hand and nervously rejecting something as "subjective" as the warding off of bad influences on the other. In most non-Western peoples the two go hand in hand. A traditional Chinese herbalist may prescribe tiger teeth for impotence, knowing full well that the patient is suffering from cross purposes and simply wants a talisman to help in realigning internal disagreement. A Western professional in mental and emotional "sciences" is not supposed to rely on such nonsense and has to work through the patient's intellect, the same intellect that is probably the main cause for the impotence. In any respect, the Juniper berries, dry or moistened, can be thrown on hot rocks in saunas, sweat lodges, and the like, and the dried crushed leaves can be used as an incense. The leaves are traditionally carried about in pouches and clothes, often the only protection or medicine carried by a Tewa Indian. Consumption of the berries or leaves is not recommended during pregnancy; the volatile oils can have a vasodilating effect on the uterine lining.

CULTIVATION: The high mountain varieties are nearly impossible to bring down to sensible altitudes and the tree Junipers are best started from nursery stock.

OTHER USES: The berries are a necessity in venison marinades and in cooking any wild tasting meat, from bear to *cabrito.* Ten berries per pound of meat is a good rule of thumb. They are also used in making sauerkraut and German potato salad. The leaves make a good garnish for fish and wild fowl, placed with the food shortly before removing from the heat.

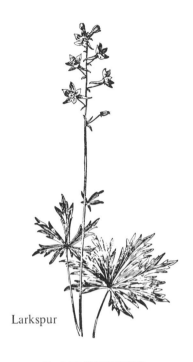

Larkspur

LARKSPUR

Delphinium spp.   Ranunculaceae

OTHER NAMES: Delphinium

APPEARANCE: The Larkspurs are showy, erect herbs with thin stems, finely or coarsely palmate leaves, and spikes of wide triangular blossoms having a pronounced backward spur. Flower colors generally are purple, blue, or violet, although several crimson species are found in California and white strains occur sometimes. The average height is two to three feet, with the plant usually in full bloom by midsummer. The seed pods are hollow and oval, with three fluted segments that split outwards upon ripening, exposing flattened dark brown kernellike seeds. Like many other plants, buds are at the tip of the stem, flowers in the middle, and seed pods below. Some plants that may be confused with Larkspur are aconite (or monkshood), with our only species having spurless blue side-flattened flowers; columbine, with five backward spurs and usually two-toned blossoms; shooting star with no spur but petals that have an extreme backward flare, also two-toned.

HABITAT: Scarlet Larkspur can be found in the Hollywood Hills and up and down the California coast, mixed with *D. hesperium* and *D. parryi,* both blue flowered. All the inland ranges of California have their own Larkspurs; nearly any area with enough moisture to accommodate Yellow Pine or Ponderosa has some Larkspur, although some may be found in sheltered areas around the Mohave Desert. In all of the forested areas of Arizona, Utah, Nevada, New Mexico, Montana, Wyoming, and Colorado the various varieties of blue Larkspurs are reasonably common. One

Arizona species, *D. amabile,* is found only in dry mesas and rocky outcroppings below 5,000 feet, adapting to the heat and lack of water by foreshortening in height, forming denser flower spikes, and having leaves that wither by late spring.

COLLECTING: The whole seed pods when ripe or near ripe, dried loosely in paper bags. Considering that no two pods are ever at the same stage in growth, all of the seeds, flowers, and buds may simply be stripped from the stems and used together; this is not as strong but may be more practical.

MEDICINAL USE: The primary function of Larkspur is to kill body lice, which it does rather efficiently. There are three ways of preparing the plant for use, all basically tinctures. The seeds (flowers) are ground, steeped in five times the volume of rubbing alcohol for at least a week, and strained. Vinegar may be used in place of the rubbing alcohol; this is somewhat less irritating but less potent. It is best used for pubic crabs. For head lice, Tincture of Green Soap, available from any drug store, is used in place of the rubbing alcohol or vinegar, and is the preferable form when dealing with this problem, the tincture forming a vermicide shampoo. The hair is moistened, the soap washed in and allowed to set for ten minutes before rinsing. For scabies, the rubbing alcohol tincture is better, but must be applied for three or four days in the evening after a hot bath or shower. Larkspur can cause rashes in some people and should be discontinued if this happens. Those terrible antilice compounds with the disgustingly inorganic ingredients can, for some people, be the only rational approach, unless the old prosaic kerosene douse seems more "organic." Less cynically, Larkspur Tincture was the old standby for much of the Western world for a hundred years and still has its place. It should not be applied where the irritation caused by the vermin is more than superficial; enough of the alkaloids can be absorbed in really bad scabies sores to make a person ill. Larkspur may not always kill the eggs so an eye should be kept out for new critters. For pets, wash with the Larkspur and green soap tincture, let set for ten minutes and rinse. Do not use if large red patches of skin have been opened by the animal.

LICORICE

Glycyrrhiza lepidota   Leguminaceae

OTHER NAMES: American Licorice, Sweet Root, Amolillo

APPEARANCE: This is a large, sweet-pea-like plant that forms large colonies connected by creeping rootstalks. The leaves are pinnate and odd numbered, with a single leaflet at the tip and pairs of leaflets along the stem, a total of eleven to seventeen in number. The entire foliage tends to be slightly sticky-waxy to the touch, often with tiny scalelike roughenings. The average height of the stalks is about two feet, with elongated flower clusters growing in the axils between the stalk and the leaf stems. The white to light yellow green, cloverlike blossoms mature into a dense cluster of finely barbed seeds, usually a half-inch long. These burred pods make Licorice, at least this species, easily identifiable, since it is the only member of the pea family with spiny fruit in the West.

HABITAT: In California it is found in rich bottom lands, in valleys, and along streams and ditches below 4,500 feet, but in the rest of the West it is a plant of the middle mountains and streams of the foothills, from 4,000 to 8,500 feet and most frequently encountered along irrigation ditches and slow-moving streams.

COLLECTING: The roots should be dug in the autumn as carefully as possible to leave the root intact. This can be a fair amount of work since the main taproots may sink three or four feet into the ground with dozens of feet of secondary shallow runners. If it is feasible, one side of a stand should be dug to the depth of at least eighteen inches, exposing the taproots and runners, then the other side should be dug similarly and as many whole roots removed from the open section as possible. As Licorice often follows along stream or ditch-side risings in moist, sandy soil, this is often not as much work as it sounds. They should be dried loosely out of the sun, which may take two weeks. The large taproots should be dried after splitting, as in Method B.

MEDICINAL USE: Licorice serves two diverse functions; it is an excellent remedy for inflammatory upper respiratory conditions, either singly or with other remedies, and it has the peculiar ability to facilitate the effects of other herbs or drugs, increasing their strength. As an example, Horehound or Mullein is more effective for early dry throat and inflamed bronchials when combined with Licorice. The other use of this root stems from its steroidal content. This is higher in the taproots, lower in the runners, and, though only present in minute quantities, can act to trigger higher levels of both estrogen and adrenocorticosteroids in cases of insufficiency. Addison's disease, an illness characterized by decreased adrenal cortex secretion, has been treated with some success by Licorice extracts in place of steroid therapy in Europe, with fewer side effects. The use of the root in the crude state, not in the form of highly concentrated selective extracts, is unlikely to have any appreciable effect, however. Chronic painful menstrual cramps can sometimes be helped by drinking at least two cups of Licorice tea a day for a week, beginning after the end of the menstrual cycle. If this brings noticeable improvement, it may be stopped after three or four months; subsequent cycles may stay less painful for a long time afterwards. If two or three months of the tea does nothing, ignore it. The root tea has often been used for treating stomach ulcers, particularly when pain is at a predictable time during the day, a rounded teaspoon of the chopped root steeped until body temperature and drunk just previous to the usual onset. Licorice root tea is strongly and distinctly sweet; for those who like the taste it is delightful, for others, an abomination. The dried smaller roots can be chewed like a confection, are loved by most children, and can be an aid as an oral placebo for those who are smokers (like myself), who are quitting (unlike myself). The tea has variable laxative effects, strong for some, feeble or inert for others, but rarely excessive or discomforting.

The presence of adrenocortical-like steroids and, according to several European studies, estradiol and estrone, make it a little risky for drinking during pregnancy. It may aggravate menopausal symptoms, but conversely it has effectively helped them, double conversely it frequently has no effect at all, so its use is a moot question. The "Licorice" candies of commerce, those disgusting rubberoid flaccid strips of childhood found in any local store pushing sweets to the usual gaggle of after school sugar addicts, contain about as much actual Licorice as present-day marshmallows contain marshmallow root—i.e., none.

CULTIVATION: The ends of the underground runners with scalelike leaf buds, still below-ground, cut eight or ten inches and planted four inches below ground in moist, well drained soil. With the right kind of growing conditions and a five-year headstart, this stout, fast-spreading plant will probably uproot the nearest house. Dig and transplant in early spring or late fall. Like Alfalfa, the roots are nitrogen fixing; unlike Alfalfa, mowing down the green part simply makes them mad and more widespread the next year.

LOBELIA

Lobelia cardinalis   Lobeliaceae (Campanulaceae)

OTHER NAMES: Red Lobelia, Cardinal Flower, Indian Tobacco, "Eyebright"

APPEARANCE: Medium-sized, upright, slender, rarely branching plants with thin, lance-shaped leaves and a long panicle of bright crimson blossoms which ripen into small seed-filled capsules. Although seldom more than an inch in size, the flowers are the most distinctive aspect—brilliant and striking and not easily overlooked. The blooms are peculiar appearing at first unless you have grown one of the garden varieties of Lobelia. The flower is a tube, branching into five lobes, the lower three fused into a lip or bib extending downward and spreading out, the other two thin and auxiliary, extending up or outward like insect feelers. Superficially resembling the flowers of some of the wild Sages, they are the only ones of their scarlet color likely to be encountered in late summer and fall. Scarlet gilia grows in drier ground, with divided leaves and regularly lobed, tubular flowers; scarlet Penstemon has a stout shiny stem, rarely blooms past midsummer, and likes drier ground, as do the scarlet Larkspurs of California, whose leaves are handlike with five to seven fingers. Texas Sage has opposite leaves and a somewhat roughened texture, preferring mountain slopes.

HABITAT: Running water and well drained muddy embankments and springs, from 3,500 feet to 7,000 feet or higher. Widely scattered in our region, and not found in the lower parts of New Mexico, western Arizona, and eastern California. The plant is listed by Jepson as occuring from the inland mountains of Los Angeles and San Bernardino counties southward, but in ten years of picking that area I have never seen a plant. If you are in California and are looking for it, check with your nearest college herbarium.

COLLECTING: Method A. The whole plant is used, chopped into one-fourth-inch pieces.

MEDICINAL USES: Lobelia is a specific herb for bronchial spasms and one of the best plant expectorants. This species is not nearly as potent as *Lobelia inflata,* the drug plant, so a scant teaspoon of the chopped plant in tea is a safe dosage. Lobelia is a stimulant to the vagus nerve and can easily produce nausea and vomiting when drunk in excess. If a teaspoon produces nausea, cut down; it is a worthy remedy for lung problems but can easily be overdone. The leaves and flowers have strong antispasmodic effects on the bronchials when smoked, and certain individuals with asthma can find it a reliable herb to smoke at the first signs of spasms. It is an effective emetic, but in those infrequent occasions when that might be necessary, Tincture of Ipecac is far safer without the stomach hangover and depression of Lobelia. As a sedative, Lobelia depresses spinal chord function excessively.

The traditional use of Lobelia by American and English herbalists seems profoundly unsafe. Samuel Thompson, the dubious patron saint of many older herbalists, created a pattern of Lobelia abuse that is still with us in such books as *Back to Eden* by Jethro Kloss. The presumption that a patient should puke his or her brains out and then take even more Lobelia is past my understanding. Lobelia in excess caused at least one documented death under Thompson's aegus. The pedantic idea that Lobelia cannot be poisonous is clearly antithetical to the facts. I know of one genial addlepate who was rushed to a hospital in Los Angeles in near coma, turning strange colors from respiratory failure, after attempting a Thompsonian "cleansing" emetic. One-half teaspoon of the official plant is a safe

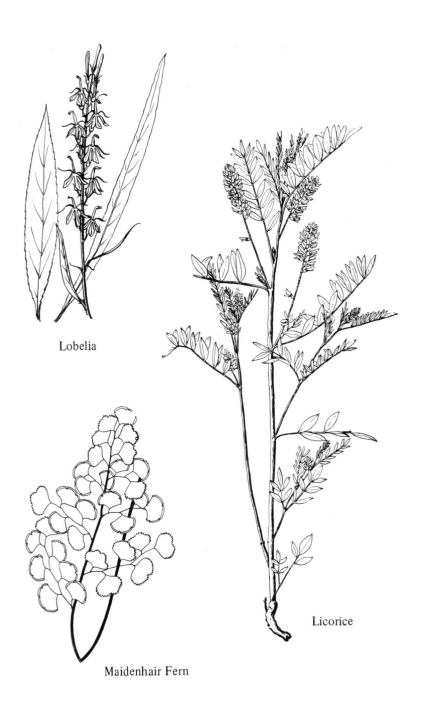

Lobelia

Maidenhair Fern

Licorice

and effective dose for lung problems. The Lobelia capsules sold in some health food stores have dangerous potential, particularly since vomiting is not reliable or quick and greater physical depression can occur. The plant steeped in vinegar or rubbing alcohol makes an excellent liniment for sore muscles.

MAIDENHAIR FERN

Adiantum spp.   Polypodiaceae

OTHER NAMES: Lady Fern, Culantrillo

APPEARANCE: A delicate fern, impossible to mistake wherever it is encountered. The overlapping fronds sprout from a creeping, scaly rootstock usually only partially hidden by mulch or moss. The stems have a peculiar polished black appearance that contrast strikingly with the round, green fanlike leaves. The individual leaflets are distinctly separated by even tinier black stems and the whole has the gossamer visage so beloved by dry floral arrangers, who make frequent use of Maidenhair. If it is fernlike and has tiny black stems, you can be assured it is one of the four species of this genera found in the West. All are interchangeable, with *A. capillus-venerus* the most widespread.

HABITAT: In our area it is found almost entirely in warm, lower canyons—wet, rocky crevices, around springs or shady northern slopes overlooking water. Rarely found over 7,000 feet, seldom below 3,000 feet except in the coastal ranges of California. Maidenhair is found throughout the world; in our range it is not predictable but is widespread nonetheless. The one place where this fern is nearly always found is the occasional narrow, precipitous canyon in lower foothills, the cooling oasis with only subdued sunlight that abounds in vegetation.

COLLECTING: Method A for the leaves, Method C for the root.

MEDICINAL USES: A remedy for upper respiratory problems and suppressed menstruation. The leaves form part of several over-the-counter cough medicines in Europe and have found their way into the folk medicine of such diverse cultures as China, Ethiopia, and Central America—a fairly reliable sign of their usefulness. Maidenhair is not a potent plant, so use at least a tablespoon in hot water for tea. Useful for sore throat, the beginning stages of bronchial infections, and laryngitis. A good cough syrup can be made by heating two parts honey, one part water, and two parts leaves (by volume), finely chopped. Powdered orange blossoms, hibiscus flowers, or ginger can be added for taste. To stimulate menstruation, one ounce of the chopped plant or one-half ounce of the root is boiled in one pint of water for twenty minutes and drunk during the day. The tea will not stimulate cramping.

OTHER USES: The dried fronds can be used in floral arrangements. Maidenhair is a widely used hair rinse, adding body and sheen. One-half cup or less of the plant is steeped in a cup of boiling water until cool, strained, and the liquid used as a final rinse.

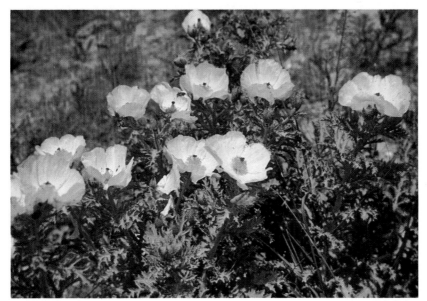

Prickly Poppy

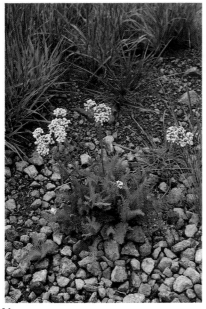

Yarrow

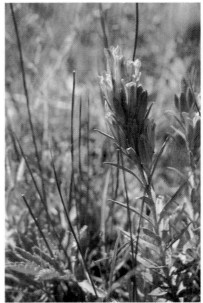

Gentian

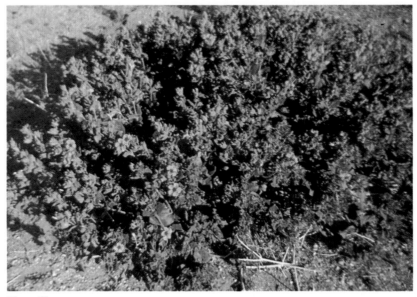

Maravilla

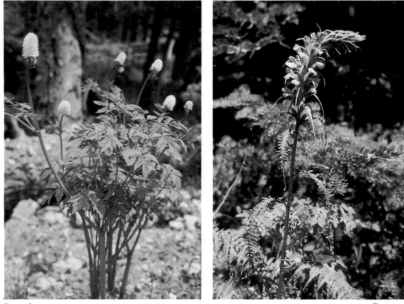

Baneberry

Betony

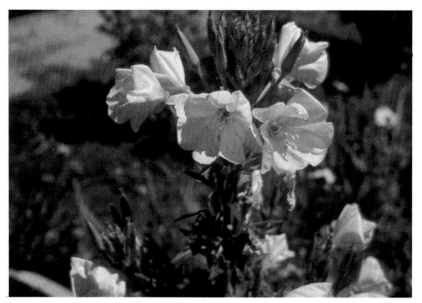

Evening Primrose

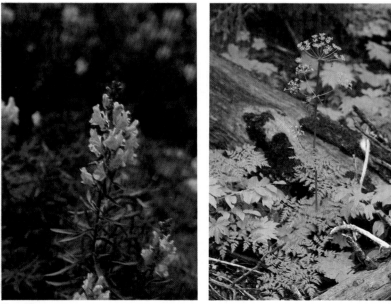

Toadflax

Oshá

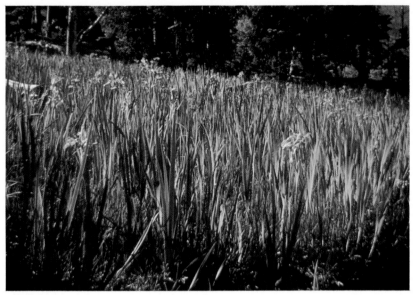

Blue Flag

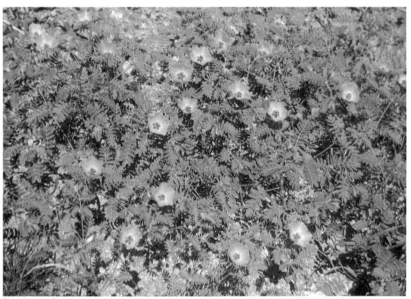

Contrayerba

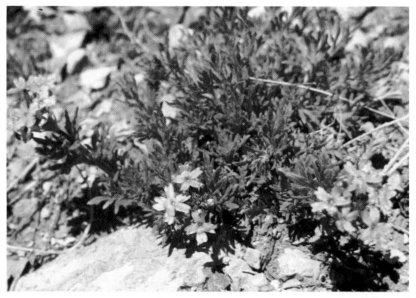

Vervain (Type 3)

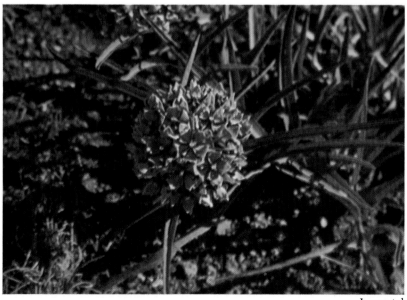

Inmortal

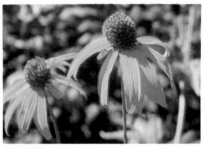
Coneflower

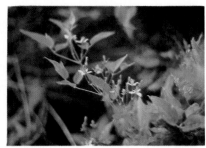
Clematis

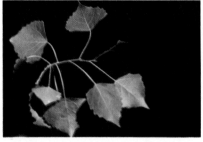
Poplar (Valley Cottonwood)

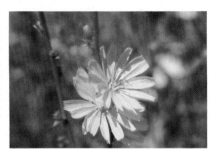
Chicory

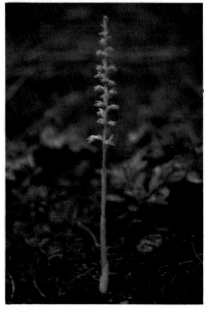
Coral Root

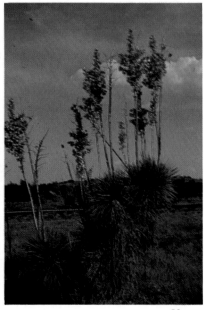
Yucca

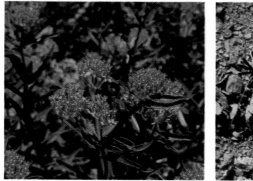

Pleurisy Root

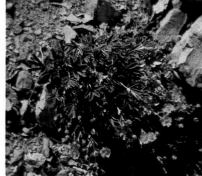

Potentilla

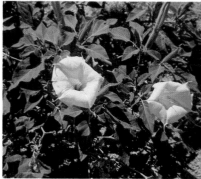

Jimson Weed

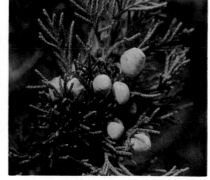

Juniper *(Juniperus monosperma)*

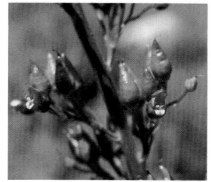

Figwort

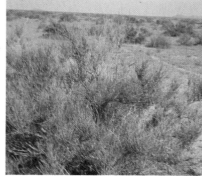

Mormon Tea

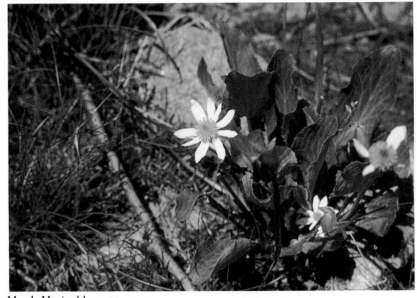

Marsh Marigold

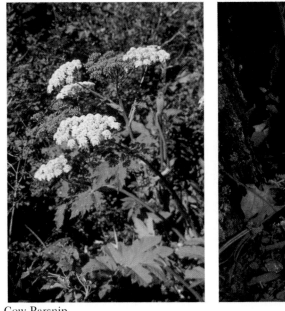

Cow Parsnip

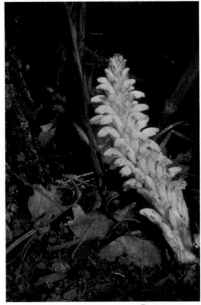

Broomrape

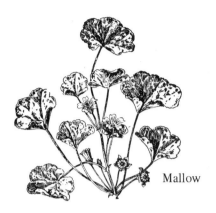

Mallow

MALLOW

Malva neglecta   Malvaceae

OTHER NAMES: Dwarf Mallow, Low Mallow, Malva, Cheese Plant, *Malva rotundifolia*

APPEARANCE: This common weed is most frequently encountered as a virtual mat, hugging the ground. In rich, moist areas it may attain a foot or more in height, long stemmed and verdant. The leaves are round, five to seven lobed and somewhat blunted palmate, the leaf stems usually much longer than the leaves and springing at all angles from the main stems. The flowers are small, five petaled, cup shaped, and from blue to white in color, clustered along the sides of the stems. The fruit is round, flattened, and resembles the wheels of cheese one so seldom encounters in supermarkets anymore. The root is light tan and rather deep. The whole plant has a slimy, mucilaginous sap when crushed between the fingers.

HABITAT: This little weed is found at all altitudes in California, from sea level in the coastal areas to 6,000 feet in the inland mountains. In Arizona and New Mexico it is encountered from 4,500 to 7,000 feet, and similarly in the mountain areas of Nevada, Utah, Colorado, and northwards. It can be found along roadsides, in old gardens and vacant lots, and in old disturbed earth in general. A weed by all standards.

COLLECTING: The whole green plant, bundled and dried as in Method once chopped into small pieces for storing. Advisable to wash well before dr rather its habitats and the downy texture of the leaves and stems combine to dusty. It is a common "marker" plant, so avoid picking in obvious or dried

MEDICINAL USES: Primarily used as a demulcent or emollient, soothing to leaves make a soothing poultice, lessening pain and reducing nerb is steeped is pleasant and green tasting, a good beverage by itself needed. Strictly sore throats and tonsillitis. A rounded teaspoon to a table ch sensitivity and in water and sipped slowly when somewhat cooled birth and as a wash palliative, but effective. The tea will help indigent and diuretic. has a mildly soothing effect upon bladder traditionally drunk in New Mexico for facil for skin irritations in infants. The tea is al

MANZANITA

Arctostaphylos manzanita, etc.   Ericaceae

APPEARANCE: The most distinguishing characteristics about the Manzanita are its smooth, matte-finished red bark and its twisted, evergreen leaves and branches. Only in the oldest plants does the bark ever shred. The heartwood of the larger branches is usually about the same shade of red as the bark. The leaves are smooth, wide, dull green, and thick as leather. The flowers bloom in little nodding clusters and are pinkish and urn shaped, maturing into red, tart, mealy berries with from four to ten seeds. Manzanita is sometimes confused with the related madrone of central and northern California (with identical use and pharmacology) and the jojoba of Arizona. Jojoba grows at lower, hotter elevations and has greenish to green brown bark. The height of Manzanitas varies from that of two- to three-foot shrubs to thirty-foot-tall individuals.

HABITAT: Although traditionally associated with California coastal mountains, Manzanita plants can be found in Nevada, Arizona, Utah, southwest Colorado, and south-central New Mexico. In fact, Manzanitas grow here and there throughout the higher foothills of our range, from 5,000 feet in the western Rockies and western slopes of the Sierra Nevadas nearly to the beaches in coastal mountains. In rich, dark topsoil below Castro Peak in the Santa Monica Mountains I have seen Manzanita trees approaching forty feet in height, flourishing in the moisture from morning ocean mists.

COLLECTING: The berries when just ripened and not yet mealy (usually April), the leaves at any time, although strongest directly after flowering. Berries, Method C, leaves, Method A. Large, heavily leaved branches can be dried singly.

MEDICINAL USES: Very similar to Uva Ursa (another, more widespread *Arctostaphylos),* it contains arbutin, a glycoside that is broken down to hydroquinone in the urine, giving Manzanita its disinfecting qualities that are so useful in mild urinary tract infections, bladder gravel, chronic kidney inflammations, and water retention. The leaves also function as a mild vasoconstrictor for the uterus and can be drunk as tea for painful and heavy menstruation. Large, frequent doses can cause intestinal irritation, as well as decrease uterine circulation sufficient to make its use inadvisable during pregnancy. An average dose of the chopped leaves is a rounded teaspoon for tea, drunk two or three times a day. Some sources consider that Manzanita is more effective as a urinary disinfectant when taken as a tincture, twenty to thirty drops in water every ~ee or four hours. Also, like Uva Ursi, a tablespoon in a pint of water makes a ๗ vaginal douche for vaginitis and can be combined with eucalyptus leaves and chᵥ leaves for a douche in cervicitis and vaginitis, or as a sitz bath after

OTₕ.

appleʼs: The berries make a pleasant, tart jelly, best when combined with or aloⁱ⁻ₕe leaves have been widely smoked either with tobacco, other herbs, for carʸ... for carⁿₑ root crowns found in the fire-resistant species have been used sufficieᵐⁱⁿₛₑ... for carⁿₑ root crowns found in the fire-resistant species have been used to brick reⁱₙg pipes, much like brier wood. Some bushes or trees have sufficieⁿₛᵉ... **CULTIVATI**carving and woodworking. The grain varies from deep yellow crowns in theₛ beautifully.

but possible, particularly when transplanting the root sandy soil. Available from some nurseries as seedlings.

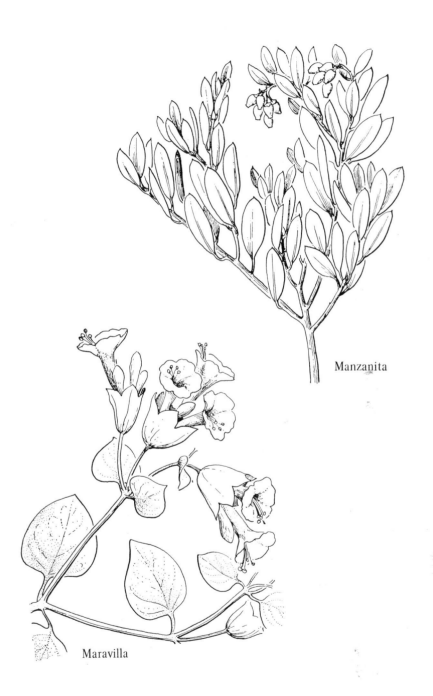

Manzanita

Maravilla

MARAVILLA

(see color plate)

Mirabilis multiflora   Nyctaginaceae

OTHER NAMES: Mirabilis, Wild Four-O'Clock, Marvel of Peru, *Quamoclidion multiflorum*

APPEARANCE: This big, attractive bush vine is in bloom for at least half the year, covered with purple or magenta flowers that open in the afternoon. They are tubular, flaring out at the ends like a morning-glory or petunia, and form clusters of three to six flowers inside a bell-shaped involucre. The leaves are smooth and heart shaped, opposite each other along the many branching smooth green stems which crisscross and overlap to form the dense mat of green and magenta found in older plants. The root is often huge (with a circumference of a foot or more), with rough-ridged brownish gray bark and a cream-colored pith flecked with what appears to be minute crystals. It has a starchy, pleasantly acrid taste that is slightly numbing and peppery after a few seconds.

HABITAT: Found on hillsides and mesas from 2,500 feet to 7,500 feet in Arizona, Utah, Colorado, and New Mexico. The comparable plant in California is *M. froebellii,* found along the drier desert-facing foothills of the Mohave and Colorado deserts as well as the eastern foothills of the San Jacinto Mountains. Not widespread but found in abundance in widely dispersed locations. It is usually hopeless to drive around or hike the back country specifically searching for the plant, but if it is late April to mid-September and the plants are present in an area, the showy flowers can be visible from a mile away.

COLLECTING: The roots at any time but most specifically in the early fall while there are a few flowers still in bloom but most have gone to seed. Try to choose plants in loose soil or on embankments, as those found in gullies and washes are nearly impossible to dig. Rare is the plant that has roots totally removable, since they can strike three or four feet into the ground. Any substantial portion remaining will regrow the next year. There is no substantial grain to the root; smaller roots can be cut and dried (Method B) and the large gnarly stumps will have to be chopped into smaller sections with a hatchet, and then cut again. Dried whole roots are tough indeed and will serve no purpose other than hammering nails.

MEDICINAL USE: Except for *M. jalapa,* the false jalap of South America, this is the only Four-O'Clock with any medicinal tradition, and there seems to be no information available dealing with its pharmacology or constituents. It is most frequently used in small quantities of one-half to one teaspoon for depressing the appetite. The root can be chewed or boiled for tea, although the first method is more effective. It is, in fact, an effective anorectic, due both to its numbing effect on the stomach lining and its mild central nervous system stimulation and mild elevating of blood sugar levels. The root is a rubifacient and local analgesic, powdered and made into a paste for applying to inflamed joints and tendons, the stomach, the chest, and even, in the case of menstrual cramps, on the small of the back. The root has strong purgative effects, one-half to one ounce of the root eaten or boiled in water, producing green, watery stools, some cramping, and immense flatulence. Although said to be used by the Hopi medicine men for inducing trance states, I cannot directly vouch for this. One to two ounces produce (besides the previous symptoms) thirty to sixty minutes of gaiety and hyperactivity followed immediately by several hours or more of befuddlement, slurred speech, and general muscular lethargy.

CULTIVATION: Small plants dug up in the fall after blooming and transplanted in loose, sandy soil.

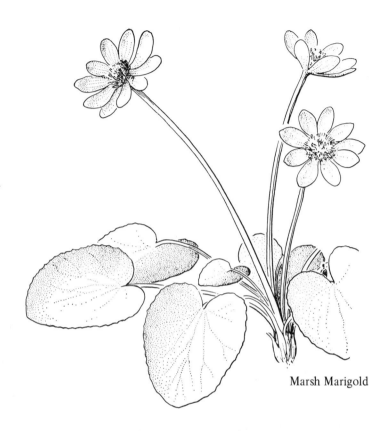

Marsh Marigold

MARSH MARIGOLD   (see color plate)
Caltha leptosepalus   Ranunculaceae

OTHER NAMES: American Cowslip, Elkslip, Horse Blobs (?!)

APPEARANCE: This little plant is quite striking, with its bright green heart-shaped leaves and white flowers with their bright yellow centers. The white "petals" are actually sepals, and are often blue veined on the underside. The yellow center is actually a colony of anthers. The flowers are bright and showy, often an inch across. The little plant is so perfect in its appearance as to border on looking plastic. The shiny leaves are nearly all basal, sometimes floating in fresh snow runoff or growing up through and melting away the snow cover. When in flower, the leaves, too, can have light bluish veins on the underside.

HABITAT: High up, from 8,500 to 12,000 feet, frequenting live streams, snow bogs, and wet spring meadows, sometimes floating in the midst of a high water creek. Found in the Sierra Nevadas from Mineral King northwards, in the high mountains of both Arizona and New Mexico, and further north. The species common in the eastern states, *C. palustris,* is encountered on occasion; it has completely yellow flowers and can attain a height of a foot or more. If it is high, and snows a lot, you will find Marsh Marigold.

COLLECTING: Whole plants when in bloom, Method A or C, depending on the size of the plants. When it is fresh Marsh Marigold can be an irritant to the skin, and gloves might be in order for those with sensitivities. Only the dried plant is used.

MEDICINAL USES: Marsh Marigold is an irritant, rubifacient, and secretory stimulant. Erratic in function, it can still be a useful remedy for some people. Small doses of a scant teaspoon or less of the chopped, dried plant once or twice a day will stimulate the flow of mucus in the lungs, digestive tract, and uterus, as well as loosen dried mucus in the bronchials and sinuses. It is an energetic expectorant without causing nausea and, combined with Yerba Santa or Grindelia, is useful in recuperation from a bronchial or sinus infection. One of the better remedies when a sinus infection has been triggered by a tooth infection in the upper jaw; a cup of tea drunk every three hours and the surrounding air made more humid. A cup of hot Marsh Marigold tea (scant teaspoon of the plant) followed by an alternately very hot and very cold shower can quickly lessen the considerable pain that such a condition can cause. The tea has some antispasmodic functions; at the same time, a hot poultice of the leaves has been of value in cases of facial paralysis. Also of use in colonic spasms and lower back pain. Care should be taken that the plant is completely dry before brewing and that large quantities are not taken or smaller quantities used for more than three or four days, since the residual acridity of the plant may cause mild kidney or liver inflammation in some individuals.

OTHER USES: The plant is a traditional pot herb, as few of its irritable properties survive heat or drying. A time-honored spring green in Europe, cooked like spinach. The scalded flower buds can be pickled in boiling hot vinegar, cooled, and used as capers.

CULTIVATION: From separated roots in the fall, planted in shade in moist areas. May not adjust quickly to very low altitude, but attractive enough to try.

MILKWEED

Asclepias speciosa   Asclepiadaceae

OTHER NAMES: Common Milkweed, Lechones

APPEARANCE: Our largest Milkweed, an analogue of *A. syriaca* of the eastern states. The leaves and stems are densely downy. The oval leaves grow in pairs, up to eight inches long. The stem is simple and erect, three to six feet. Coarse and conspicuous, it bears round balls of showy pink flowers. All parts ooze milky sap when injured.

HABITAT: In California from sea level to 6,000 feet, generally in valleys and along streams. From 5,000 to 9,000 feet in the mountainous areas of the West. Frequently encountered in undrained depressions along roads. It is widespread but erratic, common where it does grow.

COLLECTING: The roots, in the fall after the big drooping pods have seeded. Forming large tuberous clusters in some plants, the roots may never exceed the thickness of the stem and ultimately disappear into nothing in others. It is best not to belabor the digging. Unless the stand is producing thick tubers it is wise to settle for thinner pieces a foot long or less. The roots dry hard and tough, so it is advisable to chop into half-inch sections while still fresh.

MEDICINAL USE: Stimulates both urine and perspiration, softens bronchial mucus, dilates bronchials, and encourages expectoration. For a diuretic, Milkweed acts to increase the volume and solids of the urine and will aid in chronic kidney weakness typified by a slight nonspecific ache in the middle back, most noticeable in the morning or after drinking alcohol. A tablespoon boiled in a pint of water, one-half cup drunk four times a day. For the lungs, a teaspoon boiled in a cup, drunk hot. Excess can cause nausea; the same physiological mechanism that will cause expectoration will also cause nausea and vomiting. Other Milkweeds with broad leaves can be used similarly, particularly Pleurisy Root, a smaller plant with bright orange flowers and clear sap. The narrow-leaved Milkweeds are more nauseating, and if ingested should only be used in small amounts. The plant and sap of all Milkweeds contain asclepain, a proteolytic enzyme that gives some rationale to the old folk remedy of rubbing the milky juice on warts. The Doctrine of Signatures (or the concept of sympathetic medicines) has led to the use of Milkweed to stimulate milk production. Indeed, it seems to have a slight effect on lactation, but the predominant effects are elsewhere.

CULTIVATION: By seeds collected in the fall and sown in early spring.

MISTLETOE

Phoradendron spp.   Loranthaceae

OTHER NAMES: American Mistletoe

APPEARANCE AND HABITAT: American Mistletoe is a parasitic plant that inhabits many trees of our area, including Juniper, Oak, and most of the deciduous species. The various kinds are typified by opposing leaves or scales, small seeds with a gluey outer cover, and foliage of an either darker or lighter green than the host plant. Growth is generally a large clump of drooping branches, with leaves either succulently oval or degenerated and scalelike, those of the Juniper Mistletoe even mimicking its host. Mistletoe is often found in the crook of limbs or junctures of branches, where it forms a "root" imbedded in the host tree. Since it has chlorophyll of its own, the main substance obtained from the host is water, unlike Dodder or Broomrape which also obtain considerable nutrients. Nonetheless, a large mass of Mistletoe can so deplete the sap available to distal branches that it may kill large sections or even whole crowns of trees. In the West, the single most common type of Mistletoe is the species found in Junipers.

COLLECTING: The whole clump, chopped into small pieces and dried, Method C.

MEDICINAL USE: This is *not* European Mistletoe (*Viscum* sp.), the Mistletoe of herb commerce. It does, however, share with the other the ability to relax nervous tension, muscle irritability, and minor spasms; one-half to one teaspoon in tea. It will increase blood pressure, usually systolic. It is not wise to use this herb very frequently, particularly if you are prone to hypertension, and a few individuals may find any quantity mildly toxic. It is a strong vasoconstrictor, and the same proportions may aid in lessening bleeding and promote clotting. It can be a useful first aid previous to medical attention, small pieces eaten fresh until help is obtained.

A certain amount of caution is advisable, since some Mistletoes and some people don't mix well, a fact especially true in using the fresh plant. The dried plant has pronounced ergotlike effects on the uterus, stimulating contractions, increasing elasticity of muscle coats, and lessening bleeding. It should actually be compared with the two plants that have been formerly used as feeble substitutes when the ergot derivatives were deemed inappropriate for certain women: cotton root bark and shepherd's purse. Oddly enough, all three of these plants contain

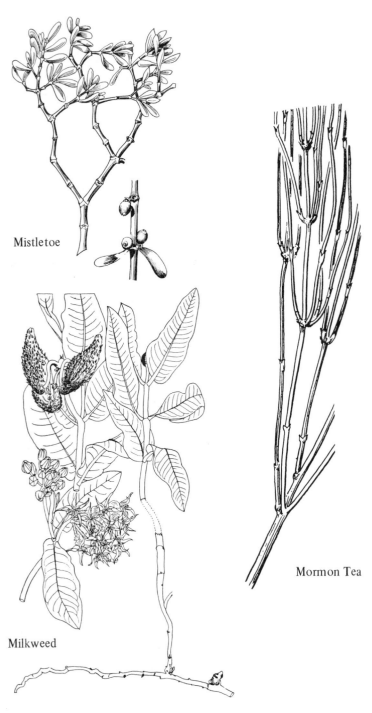

Mistletoe

Mormon Tea

Milkweed

physiologically active amounts of acetylcholine or related substances. Unfortunately, there is no reliable information on safe oral doses for use in childbirth, either from traditional Indian use or clinical use. When an herb or drug has effects on the mechanisms of childbirth it is never safe to rely on nonpregnant doses as a standard for their use in the highly potentiated state of parturition. Further, the effects of crude and refined drugs on uterine activity often vary amongst women of different races. Blue cohosh has had a long history of reliability when used by Indians of the eastern part of the country, particularly when Indian women have had to deal, intentionally and (especially) otherwise, with giving birth to infants with Anglo blood and an often excessive birth weight. Its use by women who are blond and blue eyed can overstimulate the sacral nerves and cause static, rigid uterine contractions. This sort of difference amongst our own species makes me very skeptical of some of the wholesale "disprovings" by pharmacologists in the earlier part of the century. Most of the plant drugs previously considered to have varying effects on the uterus were rejected out of hand because they produced little or no effect upon the excised uterine muscles of guinea pigs.

MORMON TEA   (see color plate)

Ephedra spp.   Gnetaceae

OTHER NAMES: Desert Tea, Squaw Tea, Cowboy Tea, American Ephedra, Whorehouse Tea, Canutillo, Popotillo, Joint Fir, Brigham Tea, etc.

APPEARANCE AND HABITAT: A small to medium-sized shrub, occasionally creeping, with numbers of jointed needles from two to twelve inches long. The overall appearance is that of a weather-beaten, long-needled, and stunted pine. The jointed stems have degenerate leaves at the nodes that are reduced to scales, either two or three depending on the species. The barkless stems range from grayish blue green with spikelike tips (in *E. torreyana*) to bright yellow green or dark green (in *E. viridis*). Some strains make striking punctuations to drab high desert valleys, with their many broomlike tufts of brilliant green. Other species virtually fade into the gravel, halfway buried by dead grasses and encountered completely by accident. Where it is abundant, as in the Great Basin, the Four Corners area, Big Bend in Texas, and the mountainous desert and foothills of south-central California, it grows in well spaced and widespread stands. The woody stems range from reddish brown in young twigs to gray and shredded in older branches. The larger branches spring from a deep rootstock, and there is seldom a pronounced center trunk. Small, exposed plants are little more than intertwined stems with a few stubby green sections, totally useless for picking. Flowers and fruit are green cones that become papery brown when dry. They bloom and mature in early spring or even late winter, and are gone by April or May. There is a reddish rust-colored pith in the center of all but the oldest twigs and branches.

COLLECTING: At anytime, even in the snow. Large plumed branches are the best, containing few of the bark-covered twigs, and are easier to process. They can be stuffed into a burlap bag or shopping bag and allowed to dry. The stems are tough and nearly indestructable except at the joints. If the tea is desired in small pieces, hang the haul in a burlap bag a foot or so above a heater or lay the bag in full sun, turning once in awhile until the stems in the center of the bag are brittle. They can then be broken into smaller, joint-long pieces by hand. It is somewhat tedious but you will have enough Mormon Tea to last you and your friends all year. There are no shortcuts. I have employed paper trimmers, paper cutters, compost shredders, and even wheat thrashers to break up the stuff. It is easiest by hand. The dark brown resinous scales that settle in the bags or cleaning area should be saved, being at least a third tannin. They make an excellent external hemostatic.

MEDICINAL USES: A distinctive, pleasant tea with enough character that many people use it as a basic beverage. Its relatives in China and India are a source of the drug ephedrine, a bronchial dilator and decongestant. Many attempts have been made to use the American plants for drug extraction but only traces have been found, not sufficient for commercial use. For our use (as a tea) it still serves a similar though feebler function. An acquaintance with a yearly scourge of longstanding pollen allergies began drinking the tea as a regular beverage to replace coffee and found that he had taken less than one-tenth his usual amount of little yellow allergy pills for that season. The decongestant effects of Mormon Tea and its subdued stimulant effects seem to point to enough ephedrine-related alkaloid content to make it functional, if not for drug manufacturing, at least for home use. The tea has a pronounced diuretic effect as well, and it forms a basic remedy for Indians and Spanish-speaking peoples of the Southwest. It can be used with safety wherever urinary tract problems occur. It had a former reputation as a treatment for the "French Disease" (syphilis), and was standard fare in the waiting rooms of "houses" in Nevada and California. It was said, apocryphally, to have been introduced by a Jack Mormon who frequented Katie's Place in Elko, Nevada during a mining rush in the last century.

OTHER USES: A tanning agent.

CULTIVATION: Nearly impossible, with its slow, tortoiselike growth and minute seeds.

MOTHERWORT

Leonurus cardiaca   Labiateae

OTHER NAMES: Lion's Ear, *Leonotis leonurus, Phlomis leonurus*

APPEARANCE AND HABITAT: This is a typical member of the mint family. The stems are stiffly square, the flat sides usually slightly concave leaving the four corners slightly ridged. The opposing leaves are deeply cleft, the upper three lobed, the lower usually five lobed, almost palmate; leaf formations are widely varied in our area. The perennial grows from one and one-half to three feet in height, with mixed lengths of stems and a scattering of basal leaves and short basal stems. The flowers form clusters around the upper leaves, and are usually white or pink. In the fall these clusters may extend a foot or more above the highest leaves in a neat segmented fashion. The only other members of the mint family found in the West with these axillary whorls are Poleo, which is strongly aromatic (Motherwort has a very slight scent if at all), and Bugleweed, with serrated but never palmate leaves. Further, the calyx tubes of the flowers are sharp and burrlike, strong enough to pierce the skin, similar to but even sharper than Horehound. Motherwort has no predictable habitat in the West, being a naturalized plant, but is encountered periodically here and there near towns and farming areas, generally between 4,000 and 8,000 feet.

COLLECTING: Method A.

MEDICINAL USE: It contains leonurine, an alkaloid with mild vasodilating effects, and the herb itself is useful in smooth muscle, parasympathetic cramps. It is most frequently employed in menstrual cramps associated with delayed menstruation which has been caused by stress or illness. It is a traditional remedy in China, used to help relax the muscles in vaginismus. It can be employed after childbirth, from the first to the fourth or fifth day, to help clarify drainage and prevent uterine infection, particularly when accompanied by an Uva Ursi or Manzanita sitz bath. If employed directly after birth it may contribute to bleeding. It has long been a home remedy in Europe as a mild cardiac tonic, particularly for tachycardia and arrythmias, although I have not observed it to have helped much at all. It is not a particularly potent remedy; a tablespoon of the chopped herb in tea as needed would be a starting place.

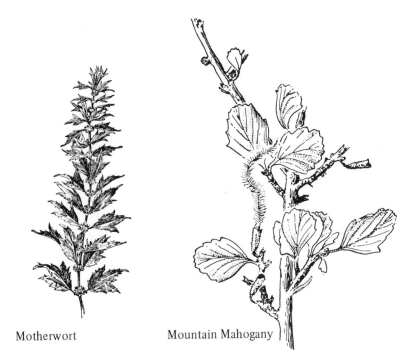

Motherwort   Mountain Mahogany

MOUNTAIN MAHOGANY

Cercocarpus spp.   Rosaceae

OTHER NAMES: Hard Hack, Palo Duro, Palo Ludo

APPEARANCE: The leaves, borne on little spurlike branchlets, resemble those of Birch. They are alternate and have a pronounced center vein with many smaller side-veins branching off. The inner margins are straight, forming a fanlike right angle, and the outside margins are sharply notched, coordinating with the side-veins. The various species have from nearly round to oval lance-shaped leaves. The bark is reddish as a rule but may be gray in some areas. The dense inner heartwood is a dark reddish brown. The flowers are small, single, and without petals, the buds starting in late winter in the axils of the evergreen leaves, the calyx forming a little flared-out five-notched tube containing numerous stamens and altogether resembling a rose without petals. The blossoms mature into a single fruit with a long feathery whip extended one to four inches, which serves both to disperse the fruit in the wind and to help it adhere in moist dirt.

HABITAT: Mountain Mahogany grows on dry, rocky slopes up to 9,000 feet and is rarely encountered in flat terrain. It is found in virtually all the mountain ranges of the West and ordinarily attains a height of six to ten feet, although some species may grow to the height of twenty feet in favored locations, with a center trunk a foot around. This is a bush predominantly of the Juniper/Piñon belt.

COLLECTING: Small branches in the spring, dried loosely, the leaves discarded. Whole leafy branches may be collected at any time.

MEDICINAL USE: A handful of the twigs are boiled for a half-hour and drunk as a laxative or as an aid in shrinking inflamed but not bleeding hemorrhoids or an inflamed prostate gland. In New Mexico the whole leafy branches are placed under mattresses to repel *chinches*—bedbugs.

MULLEIN

Verbascum thapsus   Scrophulariaceae

OTHER NAMES: Velvet Plant, Blanket Leaf, Candlewick, Punchón, Gordolobo

APPEARANCE: Mullein is a distinctive plant wherever it is found and, like Burdock and Evening Primrose, is generally a biennial. The first year the plant forms a rosette of large basal leaves and a light-colored taproot. The second year the single thick flower stalk is formed. All parts of the plant are densely hairy and flannellike, with the yellowish sap forming small blackish splotches where it has been bruised or pierced by insects. The single phalluslike stalk is completely covered with tight little flower buds, small yellow flowers, and round tiny-seeded pods, all intermixed. Some plants may form several flowering branches if the season is long or insect attack has stunted the main stem, but such plants are an exception. The normal two-year cycle is variable in lower warm or higher cold altitudes; some individuals may be annual or survive three or four years.

HABITAT: Elsewhere Mullein is a plant of waste places, but in the West it has found a solid nitch in the areas between the Juniper/Piñon and Ponderosa belts, blanketing roadsides and disturbed earth. In California it is more common in the inland ranges, forming sporadic stands in the San Bernardino Mountains and Sierra Madres, but found only infrequently in the coastal ranges and Sierra Nevada foothills, generally above 4,500 feet. Mullein is common but intermittant in the central and northern parts of Arizona and widespread in the Rockies and other ranges of the inland West.

COLLECTING: The large basal leaves of the second-year plants are preferable; they must be washed well, squeezed out, and dried by Method C. If being dried for smoking, the stems should be cut away before drying; otherwise, the leaves are dried intact and crushed for tea. The flowers and buds should be removed singly while still fresh in whatever manner seems appropriate. It is a time-consuming job and the lazier picker may treat the stalks like corncobs, slicing off the flowers, buds, and pods in a rape-and-pillage fashion. Being a trifle fussy (and purer of heart) I pluck them out singly with a pointed grapefruit spoon left over from my California years, delicately prying them out with the spoon tip and my thumb . . . a sort of Mullein-flower yoga. Although it might seem easier to simply uproot a whole plant and gut it later at a more appropriate time, this allows the plant to draw in its sap to the thick stem. Flowers and leaves subsequently removed will be substandard. Leaves should be removed in the field although the flowers may be removed from lopped off spikes within the same day. The roots are sliced and dried as in Method B.

MEDICINAL USE: Mullein is an herb for the lungs and throat and can be consumed in any rational quantity needed, being basically free of toxicity. It is a mild sedative to the lungs and is especially useful in the initial stages of an infection, when there is a mild fever, a raspiness in the throat, and a hot, dry feeling in the chest. Its effect decreases when the infection is broken and an expectorant is needed. A tablespoon of the slightly disagreeable leaves, well crushed, is steeped in sweetened water and drunk slowly during the day. The flowers are far preferable for a more energetic infection, relaxing bronchial spasms and acting as a mild sedative. Boiling water is poured over five to ten of the flowers and steeped for at least ten minutes, drunk slowly, and repeated as often as needed. People with strong skin sensitivities should take the trouble to filter the tea through a fine cloth—especially the flowers, since the coarse hairs can cause irritation to the throat membranes. Most individuals find this no problem, but people with many allergies might react to the flowers; this is noticeable immediately, causing a slight reflex contraction of the throat.

The chopped leaves have been smoked for centuries to relax spasmodic coughing in chest infections and asthma, and can be used with Lobelia or Jimson Weed for greater effect. A useful earache oil can be made from equal volumes of the fresh flowers and olive oil, steeped over the water heater for several weeks and strained. This can be warmed slightly, then several drops placed in the ear canal, which will be found especially useful for small children and pets with ear mites. The root is also a diuretic and urinary tract astringent. One-half teaspoon in one-fourth cup of water drunk before retiring will increase the tone of the triangular base of the bladder (the trigone) and aid in preventing bed-wetting or incontinence.

CULTIVATION: From the tiny ripe seeds, sown anywhere in the fall. Mullein is a useful and safe remedy but is not always common, particularly in California, so cultivation or wild sowing might be appropriate.

OTHER USES: Although not comparable in luxuriance to two-ply scented bathroom tissue, it is sort of floral designed, and may be used similarly . . . and there is no chance of confusing it with poison oak.

NETTLE

Urtica spp.   Urticaceae

OTHER NAMES: Stinging Nettle, "(expletive deleted)"

APPEARANCE: Most people know Nettles by experience or reputation, but rather few by appearance. The stems are square and substantial, with little hairs all along the length, particularly in the corners. The leaves are luxuriant green with subdued but pronounced veins, the undersides often lighter and with stinging hairs along the central vein in some species. The leaves usually come to a tapering point and are strongly toothed. The flowers are inconspicuous green, becoming small green seeds that droop from the upper leaf pairs at the stem in close clusters, frequently in such profusion as to nearly cover the stems. Where Nettles are growing in a stream gorge or steep moist embankment they can form stout fences with stems as much as an inch thick, only leafing towards the top of the plant. Such groups are virtually impenetrable. More frequently they form rich green stands of three to four feet in height. With their square stems, opposite leaves, and growing habits, they are often mistaken for large mints.

HABITAT: In the West, Nettles are always associated with water and a fair amount of moisture; along streams, valleys, marshes, and damp spots in the mountains. From almost sea level to 10,000 feet; more common above 4,000 feet.

COLLECTING: Method A—with gloves! The best time to collect for leaves is at first flowering, usually late June to the end of July. The formic acid in the hollow stingers is rendered harmless by drying or cooking, but the hairs are stout enough in large plants to still pierce the skin, so gloves may be appropriate even then. The seeds are easily collected by cutting the fruiting tops of the plant in later summer, bundling, and hanging over newspaper to dry. The seeds fall away as they dry.

MEDICINAL USE: Astringent and diuretic. The tea can be used for internal bleeding, such as excessive menstruation, nosebleeds, and capillary bleeding from heavy coughing and vomiting. An injection of the tea is a traditional European treatment for vaginitis and bleeding piles, accompanied by drinking of the tea. Nettles are a widely used diuretic, although somewhat irritating to the kidneys if used for long periods. Best used as part of a mixture or occasionally for water retention. The phosphates in Nettles help to increase urine acidity. A useful "Spring Tonic" in mountainous areas of the West where seasonal changes in diet and metabolization warrant one. (Such tonics seldom seem appropriate in places like Tucson and San Diego.) The seeds are an excellent lung astringent, particularly useful after bronchitis and such, to return tone and capillary strength to the bronchial mucosa.

OTHER USES: The seeds, because of the oils and traces of formic acid, make a good scalp conditioner and growth stimulant to the hair. One teaspoon is soaked in a cup of hot water until lukewarm (approximately twenty minutes), the tea used as a final rinse after shampooing. The fresh leaves can be boiled in a slightly larger volume of well salted water for ten minutes and the tea used to curdle milk in the making of cheese. The amount varies with the type of milk and the hardness of curd desired. The leaves are an excellent pot-herb, losing their stings upon cooking, and may be prepared like spinach or used in soups.

CULTIVATION: . . . ?

OAK

Quercus spp.   Fagaceae

OTHER NAMES: Live Oak, Fendler's Oak, Gambel's Oak, Encino, Encinillo, etc.

APPEARANCE: The Oaks of the West vary immensely in the shape of leaf and size of the plant, ranging from scraggly, shrubby Live Oaks to the archetypical Oak Tree, with most species forming both trees and shrubs, dependent upon the locale and the growing conditions. The one common feature to all species and forms is the acorn fruit. Even in the middle of winter acorns or the empty cups can be found on the plants. Most oaks shed their leaves in the fall but the Live Oaks retain them all year round, although even Live Oaks will shed in cold winters in some locations. The leaves can vary from wavy to cut leaf to deeply indented to smooth and oblong; the only reliable feature is the fruit.

HABITAT: Some kind of Oak grows throughout our range. Live Oaks often form dense thickets in foothills, with the tree forms most frequent around some moisture,

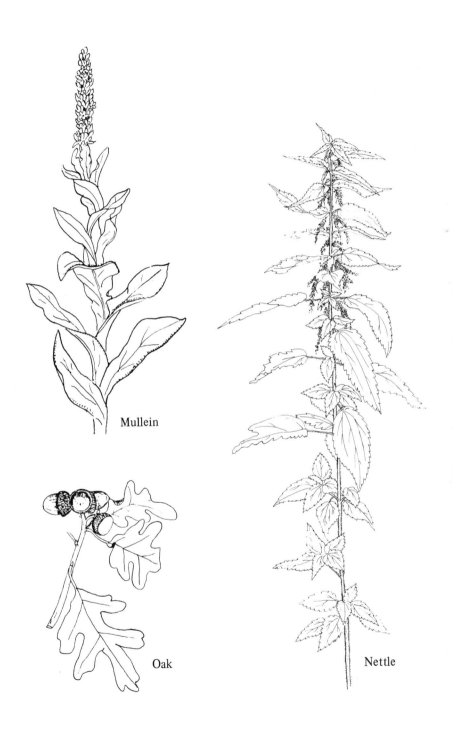

Mullein

Oak

Nettle

particularly in mountain ravines where there is moisture below ground from higher runoff.

COLLECTING: The bark is collected in early spring or late fall when the tannin is highest. The galls of the twigs when they are still flecked with red and moist, the leaves in early fall. Bark, Method D; galls, Method B; leaves, Method A, or whole branches dried singly. In small Oaks, the stems are used.

MEDICINAL USE: *The* basic astringent. A tea of the bark can be used with success as a wash for gum inflammations, as a gargle for sore throats, as an intestinal tonic, and for diarrhea. The active ingredients are tannin and quercin, the latter with similar effects to salicin. For diarrhea, the most effective mode is a tablespoon of the bark boiled in a pint of water, the liquid cooled to body temperature and used as an enema. When drunk as tea, the tannin tends to bind with substances in the intestinal tract and only a small portion survives to act as an astringent in the colon. Although somewhat outmoded in clinical practice, tannin (from the bark or twigs) is still a useful treatment for first- and second-degree burns, acting as a binder with the proteins and amino acids of the weeping, burned tissue and rendering them more impervious to bacterial action. All parts of the Oak are similarly useful as a first aid in inflammations, abrasions, and cuts, having a clotting, shrinking, and antiseptic effect. Oak should be placed first on any list of native remedies for hikers and backpackers. It is common, easily identifiable, easy to use, and effective for most of the potential problems faced in the wilderness. The leaves can be chewed into a bolus and applied to insect bites to reduce the swelling, and a piece of the bark can be chewed to lessen the pain from a minor toothache. The galls are growths found along the twigs of many Oaks, most frequently the evergreen varieties. Certain wasps lay their eggs in the twigs, and the larvae secrete an enzyme that causes the plant to form "oak apples" around them. These galls contain two or three times the tannin of the bark and are especially useful, fresh or dried, as an external wash and dressing. The quercin contained in the bark makes it a useful adjunct to bioflavenid ("Vitamin P") therapy for reducing capillary fragility.

CULTIVATION: Too common to bother with, outside of nursery stock. The scrub varieties are unattractive and the trees are slow growing.

OREGANO DE LA SIERRA

Monarda menthaefolia   Labiateae

OTHER NAMES: Wild Oregano, Bee Balm, Oswego Tea

APPEARANCE: The leaves are light green, smooth, and opposite on square stems. The leaf tips have a slight upward curl and tend to have purplish veins when in bloom. The blossoms appear as a single puff at the end of one and one-half to two foot stems, although two or even three flower balls may be found on a single stem in open meadows at higher altitudes. It is easily mistaken for a true mint; only its strong oregano scent and habitat make it distinctive before blooming. It flowers from mid-July to mid-September, with mature and immature stalks intermingled.

HABITAT: Arizona, central and northern New Mexico, 7,500–9,000 feet. Found in moist canyons, forest clearings, the fringes of meadows, and slight raised clearings above and below roadsides. The same species can be found in lower altitudes east of the Rockies but its scent is that of a lemony mint; it is occasionally found amongst the oregano-scented race.

COLLECTING: Can be picked anytime; strongest when in flower. Leaves, Method A, flowers, Method D.

MEDICINAL USES: An effective diaphoretic, particularly the flowers. Of some use in suppressed menstruation, and sufficiently antiseptic and anesthetic to make a gargle or slowly sipped tea for a sore throat. (Three to four flower heads or a tablespoon of crushed leaves.) To stimulate sweating and for sore throat drink hot, for menstrual stimulation drink cool. A mild stomachic for gastritis and indigestion. A feeble diuretic.

OTHER USES: As a spice, obviously. The flowers are rather hot and make a nice addition to salsa or chili dishes. The leaves can be used interchangeably with Mexican or Greek oregano.

CULTIVATION: Best started from trailing roots dug up in late fall but also possible from seeds picked in fall after the blossomless puff has faded in color. It likes rich, mulchy soil, a fair amount of shade, lots of moisture. It does best around bushes and under trees; single plants do poorly. Seeds are tricky, but should be sown before first snow and lightly covered with peat. Difficult to grow at low altitudes.

OREGON GRAPE ROOT

Mahonia (Berberis) repens   Berberidaceae

OTHER NAMES: Holly Grape, Rocky Mountain Grape Root, Creeping Barberry, Yerba de Sangre

APPEARANCE: The leaves of this ground cover Barberry are pinnate, usually with seven or nine leaflets in pairs along a thin but tough stem. They are rough textured, wavy margined with somewhat prickly edges, and darker above than below. The main stems seldom rise more than an inch or two, and are actually not so much stems as the upper extensions of the many creeping thin roots that form interconnected colonies. The evergreen leaves turn red in the fall, hence the Spanish name, "Herb of the Blood." The blossoms are tight yellow clusters blooming in spring, ripening to dusty dark blue berries that are bitter and slightly sweet. Both the stems and roots have a bright yellow pith color and are intensely bitter, owing to the presence of the alkaloid berberine.

HABITAT: Neither this nor the northern Pacific species is found in southern California, but it is common in all the coniferous forests elsewhere in the West, in and above the Ponderosa belt, growing on mild slopes in pine mulch and loose, rocky outcroppings.

COLLECTING: The roots and main stems at any time, dried loosely in a paper bag and broken up afterwards.

MEDICINAL USE: Identical to Barberry in nearly all respects, at least quantitatively, but seemingly more effective in cases of liver malfunction of a constitutional or chronic nature, and externally for staph infections. Also, unlike Barberry, it seems to exert a mild stimulating influence on thyroid function.

Botanically, *M. repens* differs from *M. aquifolium* and *M. nervosa,* similar plants often found alongside it in the Pacific coast states north of our range; they have stems of one or two feet in height, thicker roots, and larger berries. These are the Oregon Grape Roots of commerce, but I have personally found our Southwest species to be a bit superior. At present, most botanists have separated the *Berberis* genus into two separate genera. *Mahonia* has prickly leaves but no stem thorns and is evergreen. *Berberis* has smooth leaves and stem thorns and is deciduous. Some

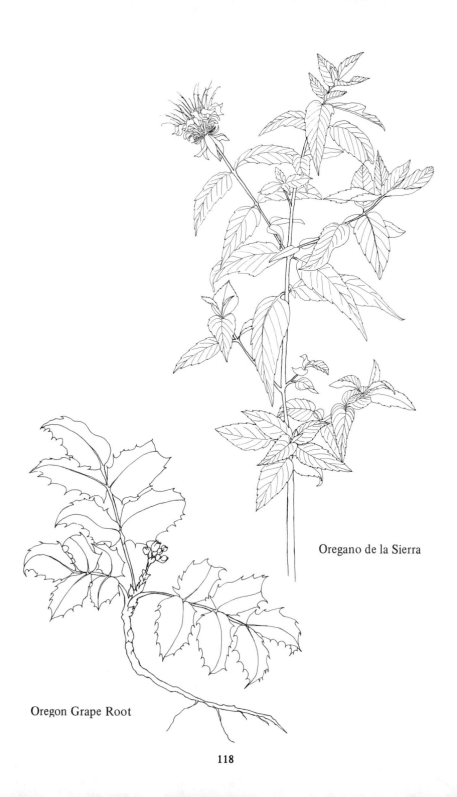

Oregano de la Sierra

Oregon Grape Root

118

botanists ignore the differentiation and still retain the single *Berberis* genus for both types. I can't blame them, considering the ever increasing muddle of nomenclature, with Latin names of a century's standing being altered and seemingly half of the doctoral candidates feeling obliged to publish some new "definitive," final, once-and-for-all clarification of this or that, as well as the publish-or-perish attitudes of some universities that demand periodic scholastic droppings from their professors. Since the original intent of Latin names was to create a universal, fixed nomenclature, it seems an unnecessary perversion to have this poor plant listed variously as *Berberis repens, Mahonia repens, Berberis aquifolium, Mahonia aquifolium, Odostemon repens,* and *Odostemon aquifolium*—end of tirade! It is still an excellent remedy, whatever the name.

OSHA (see color plate)

Ligusticum porteri   Umbellifereae

OTHER NAMES: Porter's Lovage, Colorado Cough Root, Chuchupate, "Indian Parsley," Bear Medicine

APPEARANCE: A typical parsley family plant with finely divided leaves, hollow stems, flat-topped umbels of seeds and flowers springing from a single juncture like an umbrella, and a strong celery or parsley scent. The root is large, dark brown, and hairy, with a yellow, soapy inner pith and a strong, distinctive celery-butterscotch scent. The large leaves, sometimes as long as two feet from stalk to tip, are primarily basal, with a few smaller leaves clasping the flower stalk. Older plants may have dozens of leaves and as many as six flowering stems, forming a large distinctive rosette in wet meadows. The flowers are white, the fruit gradually ripening into fennel-sized double seeds with a pleasant "celery soup" flavor. The root system in large plants can convolute and regrow in endless configurations with enough bulk from one plant to fill a bushel basket or more.

Now comes the problem: the confusion of identification. Start at 10,000 feet. Books say it grows from 6,500 feet, but I have never observed it below 9,000 and never below 10,000 feet in any quantity or size. If you are way up in the mountains and think you see Oshá, look at the seeds—those in the center are the most mature. And if the plant is at least two or three feet tall, but the seeds have little thin bracts reflexed downward it is not Oshá, but hemlock parsley *(Conioselinum)*. The root is smaller, somewhat convoluted, dark brown but not hairy, with little scent, whereas Oshá stinks! It is not toxic, however. Poison Hemlock *is,* and it looks very much like Oshá but never grows above 7,500 feet. It smells slightly fetid, like a dead mouse, and all of the stems have purplish splotches just above ground level. The root is turnip colored and hairless. Water hemlock can grow as high as 9,200 feet, but the leaves are much coarser, resembling a combination of celery and marijuana. It always grows in or right next to water and it too has a hairless, turnip-colored root. The leaflets are saw-toothed and strongly veined, with each side vein ending in the notch of the tooth, not the tip. The plant is virulent dark green. I am not trying to belabor a point, but nearly half the specimens I have seen in university herbariums labeled *Ligusticum porteri* were actually *Conioselinum* and I have at least once been offered quantities of Oshá root for purchase when the picker had mistakenly dug water hemlock roots, a deadly poison. Even the Spanish New Mexicans make mistakes, for one little valley is blithely labeled "Oshá Canyon" on all maps, but is crawling with . . . *Conioselinum.*

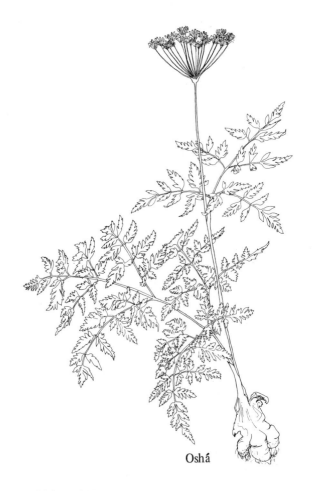

Oshá

HABITAT: Idaho and Nevada (small plants), Montana, Wyoming, Colorado, New Mexico as far south as Sierra Blanca, Arizona as far south as Mount Graham and reportedly even to the Chiricahua Mountains. A very similiar plant, *L. grayi,* slightly smaller with similiar brown hairy roots, is found in the higher elevations of the Sierra Nevadas of California, from Tulare County northward. The pickable plants start at 9,000 feet, most frequently in Aspen groves. less seldom with conifers. The largest and strongest plants grow in subalpine meadows and old burns and logging cuts, always below timberline. The biggest stands I have seen are in southern Colorado, the Wind River range of Wyoming, and Taos County in New Mexico, but if you are high enough and the land is still higher above you, you will probably find the plant.

COLLECTING: Preferably after seeding in September, but before the leaves have died off. The largest plants start to die back first and are easier to spot because of their yellow leaves. Because of the size of the roots, I have found a nurseryman's shovel and a pry bar the best tools. If digging in Aspens you will be fighting their shallow roots, so avoid them if you can. Because of their dark bark the roots can be dried in the sun. It takes a few days, but they will not rot or mildew, no matter how large; the oils render them resistant to bacteria and mold. They can be stored for years.

MEDICINAL USES: Legion. One of the best treatments for viral infections, either tinctured or chewed; brings about thorough sweating and elimination of toxins, especially if used at the first signs of infection. Up to a teaspoon of the tincture or a piece of the root the size of a walnut, every three or four hours. For sore throats and bronchial inflammations the root in any form will soothe and anesthetize almost immediately, with expectoration. Oshá makes an excellent cough syrup. One method is to grind up the root and steep twice its volume of honey over a low heat for an hour, then press out when partially cooled. Another method is to add one part of the tincture to three parts White Pine Compound Cough Syrup (a nonprescription cough medicine available from most drug stores). The tea is an excellent stomach bitter for indigestion and recuperation, especially when there has been vomiting. The tincture or tea is antibacterial and can be used for abrasions and superficial infections. Contains a number of substances only partially water soluble, so maximum benefit is obtained from chewing, tincturing, or encapsulating. An almost identical plant, *L. wallichii,* is used clinically in China for lowering blood pressure, inducing uterine contraction, and slowing postpartal bleeding. It contains volatile and fixed oils, a lactone glycoside, an alkaloid ($C_{27}H_{37}N_3$), phytosterols, saponins, and ferulic acid.

OTHER USES: The seeds and leaves hold their flavor on drying and make an excellent cooking spice, particularly in meat and vegetable combinations, with a flavor a cross between celery, parsley, and chervil.

CULTIVATION: Almost impossible. Even in northern New Mexico (elevation averaging from 6,000 to 8,000 feet), where it is most widely used, the people are not able to cultivate it for their own consumption. *Angelica pinnata,* a coarser plant of the same family with somewhat similiar functions, is grown as Oshá del Campo; the other, Oshá de la Sierra, is picked in the mountains and brought down.

PENNYROYAL

Hedeoma oblongifolium   Monardella odoratissima   Labiateae

OTHER NAMES: American Pennyroyal, False Pennyroyal, Poleo Chino, Wild Bergamot, Coyote Mint, Dwarf Pennyroyal, Dwarf Thyme

APPEARANCE AND HABITAT: These two plants are dissimilar in appearance. The *Hedeoma,* the more common of the genera in our area, is a native of Arizona, Colorado, and New Mexico. Except for the American Pennyroyal of commerce *(H. pulegioides)* found in the eastern states, the whole genera is primarily native to the central Southwest and northern Mexico, found in dry arroyos from 3,000 to 7,500 feet, or as high as the Ponderosa belt. A small, dwarf plant, it bears superficial resemblance to thyme, with small opposite leaves and many straight unbranching six-inch stems radiating from the root like a delicate pincushion. The flowers are no longer than the quarter-inch leaves and form loose clusters of two or four flowers all along the little square stems. The many dead flower stems of the previous year, with their gray dead flower tufts, are a distinctive aspect of this dwarf mint. The flowers are bright magenta, and bloom from May to late September. The plants may form two or three stems in the first year or several hundred stems in old plants. Although a fairly common plant in the drier canyons of higher ranges in northern Arizona and the Rockies, it must be looked for with a sharp eye and much patience. It took me three months to find my first plant (east of Santa Fe), but once I had formed the visualization and knew its habits, I have seen hundreds of stands in three states.

The other Pennyroyal is predominately a California genera, reaching as far east as the highest peaks in northern Arizona, and as far north as Washington and the northern Rockies. *M. odoratissima,* like the previous species, is the dominant form of a widely varying family that takes slightly different forms (and botanical names) in every foothill or mountain range in which it is found—Jepson lists thirty-eight species and varieties in California alone. The basic form is that of a group of square stems, seldom more than a foot high, with distinctive lavender or purple terminal flower puffs. The stems are usually slightly downy, with oval to lance-shaped, opposite dark green leaves, light underneath and widely spaced on the stems, all emanating from a single root. The plant, like the previous *Hedeomas,* is strongly aromatic, very similar to the traditional Pennyroyal scent, with a tinge of citrus or camphor. Larger plants may be found along embankments or mild slopes, often tucked under larger bushes, and are generally difficult to locate. Perennials such as this species' often have dead stems and flower balls intermingled with the live growth, making them a little easier to find than the ephemeral annual species. These latter types may neatly fill a hollow with hundreds of plants, but a single tiny plant may also be encountered under a bush in a gorge with no relatives in sight for miles. The distribution is from nearly sea level in the coastal ranges to 11,000 feet above Flagstaff, but this Pennyroyal can frequently be spotted along the high ridges of mountains no matter what their altitude.

COLLECTING: Method A.

MEDICINAL USE: The *Hedeoma* species contain the same volatile oils as the official species *(H. pulegioides),* and the *Monardella* is similar enough to be interchangeable. A tea of the whole plant is an excellent diaphoretic in the first stages of a cold when a fever is present, helping to relieve elevated temperatures and toxins through sweat. A rounded, teaspoon of the chopped plant is usually a sufficient dose, repeated several times two or three hours apart. The tea is a traditional stomachic for small children suffering from colic or stomach ache, in one-half teaspoon doses in a small amount of water. It is both slightly bitter and anesthetic to the stomach mucosa. Often useful where there is nausea or vomiting in children or adults, drunk after each regurgitation until spasms cease.

Part of the volatile oils, pulegone, acts as a uterine vasodilator, and larger quantities of the tea, from a generous tablespoon to one-half ounce, steeped in an appropriate amount of water, is a sure and safe menstrual stimulant, particularly when the period has been delayed several days with feelings of bloated expectations or it has become scanty and painful. Of all the usual vasodilating or irritant abortives in herb traditions, Pennyroyal is the only safe one. The uses of tansy, rue, blue cohosh, mugwort, and such, carry with them too many primary and side effects. As an abortive, Pennyroyal should be used within the first four weeks after fertilization. Up to an ounce of the herb can be drunk in a day, accompanied by one-half cup of brewer's yeast. Traditionally, if cramps or spotting occurs, this may be repeated again the second day. If the Pennyroyal is successful, a pelvic examination should follow to rule out complications. Because of the differing potencies of the various types, there is a potential for lethargy and dizziness when the plants used are high in oils, and if this occurs the dosage should be decreased. Actually, Pennyroyal is seldom effective more than a quarter of the time, and, as in any substance used to induce a miscarriage, bears with it the potentiality of difficulties if the pregnancy is subsequently carried full-term. It should rationally only be tried when a therapeutic abortion is intended, anyway. At the risk of sounding pussyfooted, I am not recommending this method, only describing its proper use, since I have encountered many women over the last decade who have made themselves very ill trying to use other, more dangerous herbs to induce a miscarriage. Further, although clinical abortions have become safer year by year and many men and women have adopted (superficially, at least) a cavalier air about them, cervical incompetence is a growing problem when an individual has had several abortions and wishes to carry a pregnancy full-term.

On the other hand, Pennyroyal can be useful in overdue or difficult childbirth, a cup or two of the normal tea sometimes helping to induce initial contractions or the diluted tea drunk, when tolerated, to clarify cervix dilations. The tea itself is quite pleasant in taste, minty and tart, and worthy for its own sake to be drunk as a beverage. As should be obvious by now, it is not appropriate to drink during normal pregnancy.

OTHER USES: The leaves and flowers of these little plants can be rubbed on exposed skin to repel mosquitoes and other biting insects.

PENSTEMON

Penstemon spp.   Scrophulariaceae

OTHER NAMES: Beardstongue

APPEARANCE AND HABITAT: This is a widely varied genera with well over a hundred species growing in the Southwest, many endemic to small areas but as a group, universal in the area. Most Penstemons are found in the middle and upper elevations and are among the showiest and most common of our mountain wildflowers. The opposing leaves are usually petioled below, clasping towards the top of the round stems, and shaped from lanceolate to pointed oval. Foliage of these middle-height, predominantly annual plants is usually smooth and waxy-glaucous. The flowers grow in various terminal configurations and are tubular, often inflated, with five lobes to the corolla. The upper two lobes often form a hood enclosing four stamens; the lower three lobes extend down and outwards with a fifth sometimes degenerated stamen sticking out like a hairy tongue. The upper leaves may completely surround the stem. These plants can be confused with the mint family (square stems) or Lobelia (alternate leaves) as well as with a number of fellow plants in the Scrophulariaceae order. Flower colors are generally crimson, purple, lavender, or blue, but don't rely too heavily on that, since some species are also yellow, white, or flesh colored.

MEDICINAL USE AND COLLECTING: The fresh herb should be finely chopped, ground in a hand mill, puréed in a blender or processer, or run through a juicer. The resultant gunk is combined with an equal volume of sweet almond, apricot kernel, or olive oil and placed in a warm place for at least a week, then strained or expressed through a cloth and heated enough to melt an appropriate amount of beeswax or canning wax in it. The whole should be poured into a wide-mouthed jar and stirred at least once before setting. This salve makes an excellent skin dressing for any irritations of the epidermis, anus, lips, and the like, both as a treatment and a preventative.

PEONY

Paeonia brownii   Ranunculaceae (Paeoniaceae)

OTHER NAMES: Western Peony, California Peony

APPEARANCE: A dense-leaved perennial with deeply and irregularly dissected basal leaves and simpler stem leaves. They are bright green or blue green and fleshy, with most dissections in sloppy threes. A large plant may become two or three feet around but seldom grows taller than a foot. The flowers are solitary in habit, drooping to face the ground as if overheavy for the stem and, although substantial enough, are easily overlooked. The thick sepals are often larger than the petals, and scalloped; the petals are a peculiar brown red or mauve color, which may extend to include the sepals, calyx, and stem, giving them a translucent purple green tint. Except for their odd color, the petals are quite insignificant and rather unlike the cultivated Peony. The roots are an extended bundle of yamlike tubers.

HABITAT: All of the coastal ranges of California from San Diego northwards and as far east as the San Bernardino and Santa Rosa ranges. It is a native of northern Nevada, Idaho, northern Utah, Montana, Wyoming, and Colorado but is completely absent from Arizona and New Mexico. In California and Oregon, its primary area, it frequents scrub oak, sagebrush hillsides, and sheltered flats but not flatlands, preferring small meadows and protected ridges in the foothills below 5,000 feet. Seldom forms dense stands but small colonies are common.

COLLECTING: The tubers, Method B.

MEDICINAL USE: Small quantities of the tea, one-half to one teaspoon of the chopped root, can be used for melancholia and those closed-cycle panic states some people get. It will also aid in scanty and painful menstruation that arises from stress or the postcontraceptive pill hormone Yo-Yos. The tea has helped orchitis and other testicle inflammations in males, one cup at night for at least a week. In prostatitis Peony can be a Jekyll and Hyde, helping immensely or aggravating the condition. It may be used as a uterine astringent in cases of excess menstruation as well. European Peony has been used as an oxytocic and abortive, but until more data on our native plant are available, either empirical or clinical, it would be very unwise to attempt its use—all Peony roots can be unpleasant in even moderate overdoses. In fact, for those with sensitive constitution or who have followed the path of a rigorously controlled diet for any length of time (macrobiotic, vegan, nonlactose veggy, raw foods, or fruitarian), no more than one-half teaspoon of the root in tea is advisable initially, as a full teaspoon might cause nausea.

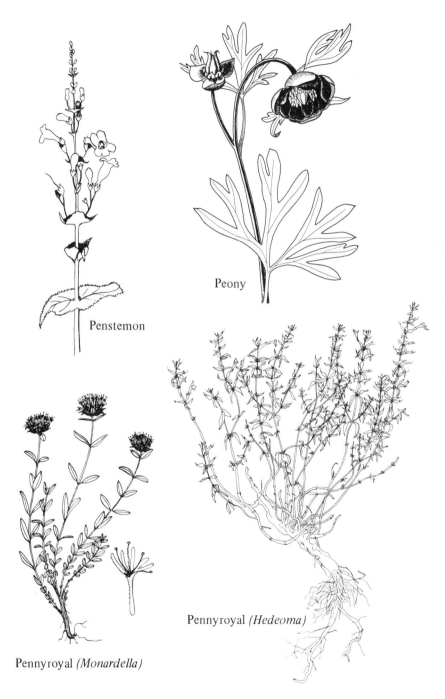

Penstemon

Peony

Pennyroyal *(Monardella)*

Pennyroyal *(Hedeoma)*

PINE

Pinus spp.   Pinaceae

APPEARANCE AND HABITAT: Two characteristics separate the Pines from other conifers such as spruce, fir, and Douglas fir. In Pine trees, the needles are in bundles of two or more with a tiny papery sheath surrounding the base of the bundles. The single exception is *P. monophylla,* a variant of the typical common Piñon of the Juniper/Piñon belts. Secondly, Pine pine cones are woody and stiffer than those of the spruces, which are papery scaled and very flexible. The cones of firs stand upright in contrast to the hanging positions of the other conifer cones, and Douglasfir cones contain little three-pointed membranous bracts between the cone scales. The various Pines are found from 5,000 feet (or lower) to, and often forming, the timberline. The little Piñon trees are the lowest in elevation, needing the least moisture, followed by the Yellow Pine and Ponderosa belts, then a whole gaggle of various Pines in the main forest areas.

COLLECTING: The inner bark, Method D, the needles collected in single branches and hung over a newspaper until dry. If the pitch is needed in any quantity, it should be melted at as low a temperature as possible and poured through a metal sieve warmed over a burner, to separate the good from the bad. The sieve may be cleaned with turpentine or may be totally unusable, depending on your tenacity. For less fussy types, the pitch may be saved as collected, adhering bark, dirt, bugs, and all.

MEDICINAL USE: Pine needles make a very pleasant tea simply for the taste, and have a mild diuretic and expectorant function as well. The inner bark boiled slowly for tea and sweetened with honey is still stronger as an expectorant, useful after the feverish, infectious stage of a chest cold has passed. The pitch is the most specific of all; a piece the size of a currant is chewed and swallowed. This is followed shortly afterwards by strong, fruitful expectoration and a general softening of the bronchial mucus. This remedy is especially useful for children. The pitch also has some value as a lower urinary tract disinfectant but would be inappropriate for use when kidney inflammation is present. In New Mexico, *trementina* (pitch) is warmed slightly over a stove or campfire and applied to splinters, glass, and other skin invaders, allowed to set, and peeled off, carrying the problem with it. While gathering near Questa one day, I encountered an elderly patriarch named Joe Rael (it was midafternoon and he was working on his third cord of wood for the winter) who had run a splinter half-way up his arm . . . or so it seemed. Cursing in obscure Spanish, he grabbed some pitch, warmed it over a cigarette lighter in a crushed beer can, and slapped it on the wound, waited a moment, and plucked out the splinter with the pitch. I tried the same thing the next week, and got a blister for my troubles. An acquired technique, I guess.

PIPSISSEWA

Chimophila spp.   Ericaceae

OTHER NAMES: Prince's Pine, Princess Pine, "Wintergreen"

APPEARANCE AND HABITAT: The three species of Pipsissewa in the West are small (four- to ten-inch) evergreen plants with shiny, leatherlike leaves in loose whorls along tough stems that arise from creeping rootstalks. The flowers grow in little open nodding clusters of exquisite blossoms that resemble the kind little children draw. They range from flesh colored to pink, occasionally white, made up of five sometimes reflexed, round concave petals, with the reproductive parts forming a broad sticky cone in the center, bright green in color. *C. umbellata* is the most common species, found throughout the northern hemisphere above 6,500 feet, including all the substantial coniferous forests of our major ranges. The stemless leaves are dark green, lanceolate, and shallow toothed, wider towards the tips, narrowing gradually until they join to the stem. Older plants will form auxiliary stems off of the main part, but these are mostly foliage with few if any flowers. *C. maculata* has an almost identical appearance, but with pronounced light spots on the leaves, and is confined, in our range, to Arizona, Utah, and probably Nevada. *C. menziesii* is only found in the Pacific states, from San Diego County northwards, and inland to the San Bernardino Mountains and the Sierra Nevadas; in Pine woods above 4,500 feet. It has white or light pink flowers with partially closed petals, and leaves that are lightly spotted and more alternate than whorled. The shape is more oval than lanceolate and the serrations are shallower or nearly lacking. All three are inhabitants of moist, shady glens and well forested slopes, growing in leaf and needle mulch. They are petite plants that are easily overlooked unless in flower. They are seldom found near roads and habitations and more likely to be encountered by the hiker or light camper with a lust for moist, secluded "forest primeval" kinds of places.

COLLECTING: The aboveground stems, dried loosely or by Method C. Leave the roots and pick carefully; these are widespread plants but slow-growing and slow to propagate and not always abundant in our mountains.

MEDICINAL USE: Similar in use and pharmacology to Uva Ursi, Manzanita, Pyrola, and Blueberry, all relatives. It is much less astringent than Uva Ursi, with a stronger diuretic action and less irritation of the intestinal linings. Pipsissewa contains ursolic acid, the glycosides arbutin, ericolin, and its own specific, chimophilin, all of which are excreted in the urine as disinfectant substances. Pipsissewa is an almost perfect remedy for kidney weakness or chronic mild nephritis, and can be taken several times a week for extended periods; it can reduce the problem substantially, given time and a reasonable diet. The average dose is a scant to rounded teaspoon of the chopped leaves, *boiled* for twenty minutes or more. In short- or long-term skin eruptions, two or three cups a day will temporarily aggravate but considerably shorten the duration of the symptoms. The fresh leaves, moistened, are an effective counterirritant, if left on for a half-hour or longer.

OTHER USES: Pipsissewa has been a traditional part of root beer and is still allegedly included in several brands.

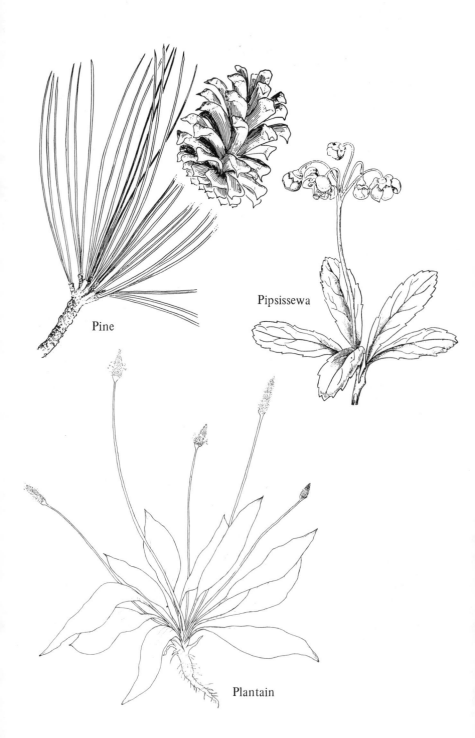

Pine

Pipsissewa

Plantain

PLANTAIN

Plantago major   Plantaginaceae

OTHER NAMES: Lanten

APPEARANCE: A common perennial weed, found virtually around the world. Highly adaptable, it can range in appearance from the ground-clasping bane of lawn fanciers (always growing just under the mower blades and seeding seemingly overnight) to the virulent green, starkly ribbed lilylike specimens found along mountain streams. The distinguishing characteristics are the parallel veins of the leaves, the strong hemplike fibers of the stems and leaves (if the stem is broken back, the fibers can be pulled out virtually intact), the completely basal leaves that flare outward from the root, and the light green brown flowering stalks that are densely covered along the tips with tiny yellow green flowers. The phallic appearance of the flower stalks has rendered it an aphrodisiac in many cultures. The leaves and roots, if rubbed between the fingers, have a slippery, mucilaginous texture. Plantain is a plant that, once identified, is always remembered.

HABITAT: Very common in moist waste places, lawns, and wet meadows and along stream beds in mountains.

MEDICINAL USES: Primarily the fresh plant. The leaves make an excellent poultice for abraded skin and insect bites. Its frequent appearance where mosquitoes are found and its proximity to water make it the basic treatment for their bites; a leaf is chewed into a bolus and placed over the bite. Proteolytic enzymes found in the fresh leaf and the fresh or dried root make Plantain useful as a gentle internal vasoconstrictor for mild intestinal inflammation, from stomach ache to dysentery and inflamed hemorrhoids. The fresh juice or dried leaves in tea can help bladder inflammations. If a juicer is available, a fine douche for vaginitis is made by combining two tablespoons of Plantain juice and a pint of warm water with a pinch of table salt. The dried leaves or roots will be found useful in treating chronic lung problems in children; a mild cup of tea (scant teaspoon in hot water) every morning. The fresh juice can be almost miraculous in mild stomach ulcers; it can be preserved with twenty-five percent vodka or ten percent grain alcohol, one teaspoon in warm water one hour before every meal until pain ceases. The seeds are closely related to psyllium seeds and can be used similarly, a tablespoon or two soaked in hot sweetened water or fruit juice until a mucilage is formed and the whole gruel drunk as a lubricating laxative.

Another common Plantain, *P. lanceolata* or Lance-Leafed Plantain, is frequently encountered in lawns and waste places. All uses are the same. The leaves are more grasslike and a darker green. It is a much less distinctive plant and should only be picked when flowering enables more positive identification. All young Plantain plants, for that fact, can bear superficial resemblances to several species of lilies and (more dangerously) to green hellebore, so it is wise to look for the flowering stalks of Plantain before picking. If it has branches, leaved stalks, or single, distinctive flowers, and if the root is anything but small and turniplike, it isn't Plantain.

OTHER USES: The fresh, streamside leaves of unflowered Plantain are a rather tasty green. The fibers should be removed first, unless the leaves are still rather small.

PLEURISY ROOT (see color plate)

Asclepias tuberosa   Asclepiadaceae

OTHER NAMES: Butterfly Milkweed, Colic Root, "Inmortal"

APPEARANCE AND HABITAT: This is a most unusual Milkweed in two respects. It has no milky sap, at best managing an opaque green juice, and the flowers are a startling profusion of orange blossoms. Although not found in California, it occurs in southeastern and northeastern Arizona, Utah, both sides of the Rockies, and the northern half of New Mexico. Because of its airborne seeds, it is very sporadic in our area but can be abundant locally. It is common in the Midwest. The leaves, unlike most Milkweeds, are alternate or indiscriminately placed in dense profusion on the thick, two-foot stems. They are lance shaped and distinctly stem-clasping toward the flowers. The many small flowers occur in tense terminal clusters with the typical backward flaring petals and the peculiar hooded crown of the Milkweed genus. The pods may be up to three or four inches long, furry, and upright. The root is medium brown, white pithed, ridged, and extending two feet or more into crevices, sometimes forming a huge knotted tuber several pounds in weight. In our area, Pleurisy root is found in Ponderosa clearings, the edges of meadows, and gullies or rocky arroyos. It is not predictable in locality or habitat and would not be noticed except for the brilliant flowers or large pods.

COLLECTING: The roots, dug like Inmortal, Method B. Large roots may need to be split with a hatchet several times before they are sliced smaller.

MEDICINAL USE: In some parts of eastern New Mexico this is also called Inmortal, and is quite similar to that plant in nearly all respects except for a lack of cardiac effects. It is a stimulant to the vagus nerve, producing perspiration, expectoration, bronchial dilation, and the like. As its name signifies, it is useful for pleurisy and mild pulmonary edema, increasing fluid circulation, cilia function, and lymphatic drainage. An average dose is a scant teaspoon of the chopped root, boiled in water, one or two cups drunk in a day. Amounts of a tablespoon or more of the root can cause nausea or vomiting.

POLEO MINT

Mentha arvensis   Labiateae

OTHER NAMES: Brook Mint, Indian Mint, Corn Mint, Wild Mint, Horse Mint, *Mentha canadensis*

APPEARANCE: A typical Mint family member; square stems, leaves in pairs, with a creeping rootstalk the main form of propagation. For all practical purposes, this is the only native true mint in the United States. Poleo (the Spanish Name) is in some ways the most distinctive and delicious smelling of all the mints, the scent a cross between Peppermint and Pennyroyal. The leaves are slightly notched, frequently downy, and, compared to the more common mints, relatively smooth leaved. The plant is light green in sunny areas and darker in shade, the height varies from less than a foot when found in back washes and dried sumps to as tall as three or four feet when encountered growing amidst thick stands of Sweet Clover or Willow. Two characteristics distinguish it easily from more common naturalized mints. First, the plant does not flower in terminal spikes as other of its relatives but in the axils of the upper leaves, the flowers usually light pink to lavender. Second, unlike other mints Poleo frequently branches, particularly in late summer or in drier

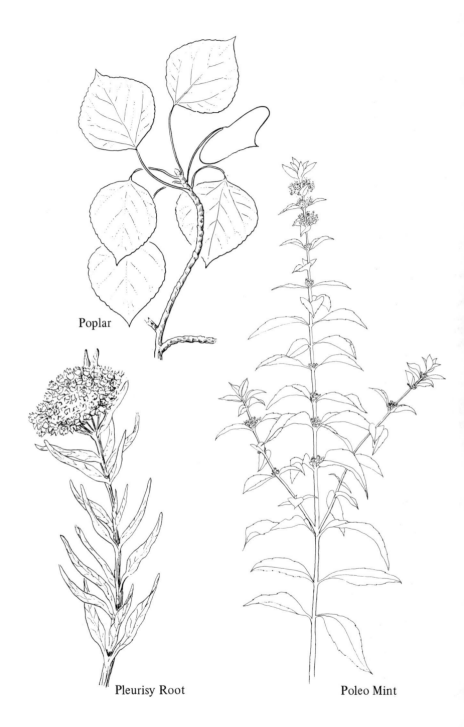

Poplar

Pleurisy Root

Poleo Mint

streams, often a dozen or more times. In other locales it can grow almost vinelike up through taller plants, its stems thin and weak, only branching when it reaches sunlight. A similar plant, European Pennyroyal *(Mentha pelugium),* can be encountered on occasion, particularly in the Sierra Nevadas and southern Cascades of California, but is smaller, with distinct woody stems and many creeping. basal stems as well as upright flowering stalks. The overall appearance of Poleo is more delicate than that of the other mints, particularly the common Spearmint, and the stems are altogether more fragile. It is a highly variable plant, changing subtly from watershed to watershed, accidentally forming a thumbnail profile of the authors of botanical textbooks. Tolerant botanists lump the whole bloody mess into *"Mentha arvensis";* nitpickers discover endless varieties and subspecies *(Mentha arvensis, var penardi . . . glabrior . . . hooplesii . . . borealis,* etc.).

HABITAT: From as low as 2,500 feet (below Lake Hughes in southern California) to 10,000 feet (Taos Ski Valley, northern New Mexico), but always along streams and running ditches or very moist meadows. A plant that is found relatively unchanged across the northern latitudes from China to Labrador.

COLLECTING: Method A. The stems are very aromatic and, unlike other mints, soft and soluble; therefore, should be included with the leaves when cut for storage.

MEDICINAL USE: Above all, a stomach anesthetic and tonic, useful for colic, indigestion, and dizziness that relates to indigestion. A tablespoon or less steeped in a cup of water and sipped slowly. Makes an excellent sun tea, brewed either fresh or dried. Poleo makes an excellent and delicious after-dinner tea as well as an aperitif in a jigger of brandy or white wine when appetite or digestion seems a bit off. The terpene pulegone is the active substance of Pennyroyal and is found in some quantity in Poleo, along with large amounts of menthol, so in addition to the stomachic effects of this mint, it also can be used to stimulate scanty or delayed menstruation, particularly if accompanied by a bloated sensation or painful cramps. Pulegone repels mosquitoes, so the fresh leaves of Poleo can be rubbed over bare skin to prevent their bites.

OTHER USES: The Japanese variety is the source of a good deal of the plant-derived menthol used in pharmaceutical manufacturing. The fresh leaves make an excellent liner for cake tins in place of grease and impart a delightful flavor to light cakes, especially pound cake and angel food cake.

POPLAR (see color plate)

Populus spp.   Salicaceae

OTHER NAMES: Cottonwood, Alamo, Aspen, Quaking Aspen

APPEARANCE: In the West, the leaves of the Poplar clan are usually heart-shaped with long stems. Leaf buds are waxy and scaled, mature leaves bright green, turning brilliant yellow in the fall. The long hanging catkins appear before the leaves; the bark is light and smooth, growing deeply furrowed in older trees. The Aspen retains smooth bark.

HABITAT: Cottonwoods and Poplars are always associated with water and Aspens with high mountains. Fremont's Cottonwood is found along live water and underground springs throughout our range; the narrow-leaved Cottonwood more specifically in Arizona, New Mexico, southern Colorado, and west Texas. Quaking Aspen grows wherever there are mountains at least 8,500 feet high, although sometimes descending to 6,000 feet or less in such ranges. Poplars and

Cottonwoods are big, substantial permanent residents, Aspens are thin weed-trees found high up in conifer burns and in unaltered ecologies, are eventually replaced by fir, Pine, or spruce. Aspens sometimes form permanent stands along subalpine meadows, covering whole hillsides like thin, white sentinels.

COLLECTING: Leaf Buds, Method C; bark, Method D; leaves, Method A. Buds should be collected in early spring, leaves in midsummer, bark in late fall or spring.

MEDICINAL USE: All of the *Populus* family contains varying amounts of salicin and populin, relatives and precursors of aspirin that are useful wherever a fever needs reducing or an anti-inflammatory is appropriate. Poplar is a safe substitute for quinine in intermittent fevers. The bark is the most effective part for tea but is rather bitter; for this reason the leaves, although feebler, are preferred by some. The various parts are also serviceable for mild urinary tract inflammations and for use as a diuretic, increasing urine acidity where that may be desirable. An excellent old-fashioned bitters can be made by steeping an ounce of the dried bark, one-fourth ounce of Licorice Root, and a teaspoon of cloves in a fifth of brandy. After a month the bitters have "matured" and can be sipped on for poor appetite, indigestion, and feverishness. Through no fault of the herbs, excess "sipping" can lead to undesirable side effects. The leaf buds, particularly in those species where they are aromatic and balsamic, make an excellent ointment for burns and skin irritations. (The buds are the most potent part of the plant but are only slightly soluble in water.) Sufficient buds to fill a jar are covered to the top with olive oil or sweet almond oil and placed in a warm place for a week. The strained oil can be used as it is or a small amount of beeswax can be added over a low heat until melted and then stored in a wide-mouthed jar for use as a salve. The fresh or dried plant can be used in fomentations or poultices for muscle aches, sprains, or swollen joints. A tea of the bark will aid in diarrhea.

CULTIVATION: From nursery stock.

POTENTILLA   (see color plate)

Potentilla spp.   Rosaceae

OTHER NAMES: Cinquefoil, Five-Fingered Grass, Silverweed, Goosegrass

APPEARANCE: To begin to describe all of the Potentillas in the southwestern mountains would be impossible. Fortunately, however, several characteristics are universal among these many species. The flowers are nearly always yellow and resemble closely their relative the Rose, with five separate petals and five green subtending sepals. The pistils in the flower center are numerous, also like the Rose. The leaves are sharply and regularly serrated like another relative, the Strawberry. Some species form five-, seven-, or nine-fingered hands, others have pinnate leaves with the leaflets equally spaced on both sides of the central leaf stem, ladderlike. The name "Silverweed" refers to the densely downy leaves of many varieties that give them a distinctly silver green color. Most Potentillas are low growing or totally basal plants, and all have a chaffy, pink-pithed taproot that is intensely astringent to the taste. Some types grow directly on the ground in high meadows, hidden in the grass, but most clump up a bit in a typical herblike fashion. The only large Potentilla of our area is *P. fruticosa* or Bush Cinquefoil, a shreddy-barked shrub with many small, showy yellow flowers and tiny thin-fingered silver-haired palmate leaves.

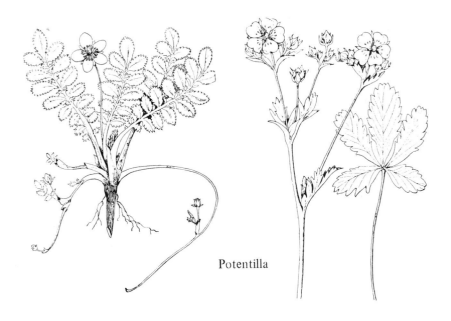

Potentilla

HABITAT: The various species, a botanist's nightmare of crossbreeding, are universal in our higher mountains, often covering the floors of high meadows and sandy flats from 6,000 feet to above timberline. Bush Cinquefoil can be found in most high mountains, most frequently from 8,000 to 9,500 feet. Potentilla is a reliably frequent mountain plant.

COLLECTING: The entire plant (excluding the bush type); root, stems, leaves, and flowers, dried loosely in paper bags and chopped finely for storage. Bush Cinquefoil, the most densely foliated stems, Method A.

MEDICINAL USE: Potentilla, like nearly all members of the Rose family, is an astringent, tightening tissues, relieving inflammatory conditions, having the strength of Oak bark, but, like Alum Root, is gentler internally. A strong tea of the plant makes a useful mouthwash and gargle for sore throat or tonsil inflammations and helps to reduce gum inflammations. When drunk two or three times a day it will speed up the healing of both esophagus and stomach ulcers or inflammations, but should be used for a week or more, depending on the magnitude of the problem. A pot of the tea will lessen fevers and diarrhea; its common distribution in the mountains makes it another plant that should be relied on for first aid when hiking or packing the back country. The fresh plant can be placed in some water and made into a sun tea for a soothing astringent lotion, applicable to abrasions, sunburn, windburn, poison oak, and the like. It will help prevent saddle sores on horses, mules, or burros. The tea is liberally sloshed over their backs when they are resting after the packs and blankets have been removed. The leaves and flowers placed in shoes will help prevent blistering when hiking.

PRICKLY POPPY   (see color plate)

Argemone spp.   Papaveraceae

OTHER NAMES: Thistle Poppy, Cardo Santo, Chicalote, Mexican Poppy

APPEARANCE: A peculiar plant, Prickly Poppy has all the superficial resemblances to a thistle; prickly leaves and stems, blue green inconspicuous foliage, and a height of one and one-half to three feet. The flowers, however, are big showy poppies with five white papery petals and a golden yellow center that bloom from late spring to autumn. Totally unexpected if you had been observing the plants before flowering, scruffy and weedy, the sort one instinctively avoids. The stem-clasping wavy leaves are from three to eight inches long and the stem is stout and well armored. All parts of the plant have a yellowish milky sap that turns black in contact with the air. The flower buds are three horned and well barbed; the flowers themselves lose their petals one at a time, to be eventually replaced by ridged pods with a tip of black sap. The blooms are in clusters, the center being the oldest, and, when fruiting, the earliest to ripen. The football-shaped pods contain poppy seeds that are milky white at first, becoming mottled brown black when mature, gradually sown by the wind as the sides of the capsules curl back. Annual, sometimes perennial.

HABITAT: From high desert plateau (3,000 feet) in southern California (common on both sides of Cajon Pass) to 8,000 feet in New Mexico, it is found throughout the Southwest. It has no typical habitat, although most common in disturbed earth and railroad embankments.

COLLECTING: The seeds when brown and before the pod has opened, the plant when in flower (Method A). Since the sap is narcotic enough that a few moments of handling the plant results in skin insensitivity to the spines, it is necessary to gather this nasty with thick gloves. There is probably some easy way to winnow the seeds, but I have not found any, except drying the pods in the sun, covering them with burlap, and stomping them to death. The seeds can then be sifted. For tea, the leaves should be stripped off with gloves and chopped up for storage. The whole flowering tops, pods and all, can be treated in like manner. The fresh plant can be juiced, stalks, leaves, and flowers, and preserved with twenty-five percent vodka or ten percent alcohol.

MEDICINAL USE: The juice of the plant has a rubifacient and slightly caustic effect; used straight for warts, diluted for skin ulcerations, externally. The fresh juice, greatly diluted, has a long traditional history as a treatment for opacities of the cornea. I can find no specifics either on dosage or clinical uses; it isn't as far-fetched as it sounds. The only standard external treatment for opacities remains a pharmaceutical preparation of the juice of fresh Dusty Miller in compound (*Senecio cineraria*). The preserved juice, with three or four parts water, can be used for heat rash, hives, and jock rot. One-half teaspoon in water in the morning for a few days will lessen the irritability of urethra and prostate inflammations. The whole plant can be boiled into a strong tea and used for bathing sunburned and abraded areas for relief of pain. The dried plant is a feeble opiate and helps to reduce pain and bring sleep, a rounded tablespoon in tea. The seeds are a strong cathartic, a teaspoon or two crushed in water and drunk. They have somewhat of a sedative and narcotic effect when eaten and have traditionally been smoked alone or with tobacco. They are quite edible, being one of our best forage seeds, but their

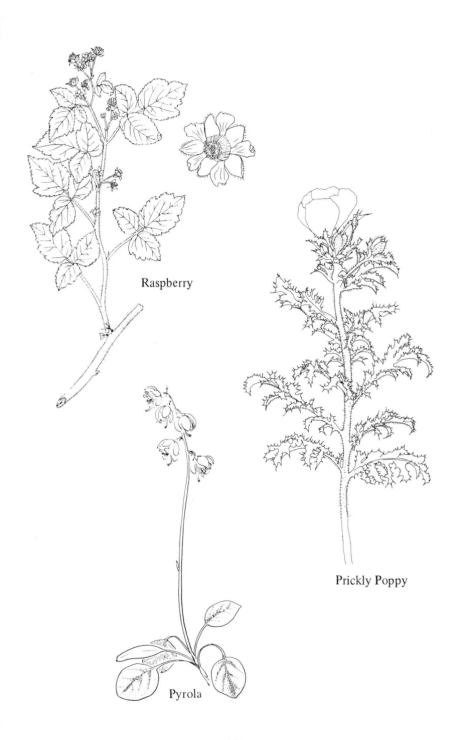

Raspberry

Prickly Poppy

Pyrola

drug activity tends to limit their ingestion in large quantities. The seed oil was formerly used in place of castor oil.

CULTIVATION: The seeds sown free in fall. Easier in disturbed slopes or embankments. Can get out of hand if not watched and thinned from year to year.

PYROLA

Pyrola spp.   Ericaceae

OTHER NAMES: Shinleaf, "Wintergreen," Round-Leafed Wintergreen

APPEARANCE: This varied little family is closely related to Pipsissewa, and is similar in appearance and habitat. Pyrola is a low-growing perennial with a thin, creeping root and shiny petioled bright or dark green leaves that are round or oval and primarily basal. The little flower stalk holds several five-petaled flowers (in one species only a single bloom) that are delicate and neatly scalloped, usually pink, reddish, or white. They have ten stamens and, flower stalk and all, are seldom taller than six inches.

HABITAT: Moist, shady places in coniferous forests or above streams; anywhere that you find Pipsissewa, Valerian, or Blueberries is a good place to start looking. Pyrola blooms from midsummer to early autumn and, unless it is in flower or you happen to be lying on your stomach under a pine with your nose two inches away from it, unlikely to be noticed, since the basal form is inconspicuous to say the least. Widespread and common but, like Pipsissewa, Pyrola prefers relatively undisturbed high forest and dislikes summer campgrounds with barking dogs, beer cans, and RV holding tanks.

COLLECTING: Due to their small size and moistness, Method C.

MEDICINAL USE: Identical with Pipsissewa and often substituted for it in herb and drug commerce. This used to bother me in a self-righteous sort of way, particularly after having to walk halfway around a mountainside to find a neat little stand of Pipsissewa . . . and probably stepping on a thousand Pyrolas in the process. In fact, however, the pharmacology of the two plants is the same.

RASPBERRY

Rubus spp.   Rosaceae

OTHER NAMES: Western Blackberry, Red Raspberry

APPEARANCE AND HABITAT: The common species in Arizona and the Rockies is smaller and more prickly, growing most frequently on moist slopes and above streams, only occasionally found as low as the Ponderosa belt. Seldom more than three or four feet tall, the stems are distinctly different for flowering growth (small leafed) and new growth (large leafed, no flowers). The flowers are cream white and the fruit is the typical Raspberry. The California species can be found along streams and in moist areas from almost sea level to 6,000 feet, and is a many-branched bush with fewer thorns and a dark purple blackberry-type fruit.

COLLECTING: For both types, the large-leafed stems or branches just before or during flowering, Method A. The roots in the fall, Method B. For obvious reasons the leaves should be stripped with gloves after drying. They tend to be fluffy and somewhat cottony and it is easier to store and use them if they are cut into fine pieces with scissors or rubbed between the gloved hands like Sage.

MEDICINAL USES: A mild uterine astringent, reliable and safe both for excessive menstrual bleeding (a tablespoon of leaves in tea every three hours) and during pregnancy to prevent spotting in the first trimester and to increase muscle tone in the uterine walls (two or three cups a day for the duration). Drunk after birth it will help decrease uterine swelling and cut down on postpartum bleeding. The leaves and especially the root are serviceable as a treatment for diarrhea and dysentery, a strong cup of tea drunk at body temperature every hour until symptoms decrease. The fruit is also useful for the same purpose. The roots and leaves can be mildly sedative for some people and the root and fruit are slightly laxative and diuretic.

OTHER USES: The berries contain enough pectin to set up nicely as a preserve or jelly, and when puréed can be boiled with honey or sorghum for a delicious pancake syrup. The syrup can also be used straight to lessen feverishness or diarrhea in children.

CULTIVATION: Difficult to transplant. It is advisable to use nursery stock.

RATTLESNAKE PLANTAIN

Goodyera repens   Orchidaceae

OTHER NAMES: Net Leaf Plantain, Spotted Plantain, White Plantain, *Peramium*

APPEARANCE: A denizen of the deep forests, this plant has several thick roots and a ground-hugging flat basal rosette of thick green leaves, intricately mottled in white. This gives it a diamondback appearance and hence its name. It sends up a single, somewhat scaly stem of about a foot in height bearing a number of small greenish white orchidlike flowers that form a one-sided raceme.

HABITAT: Rattlesnake Plantain is only found in rich forest areas, off the beaten path in the shade of deep conifer stands. Its habitat is from 8,000 to 10,000 feet, although in very sheltered areas it may descend to 7,000 feet. Although not found in southern California it is fairly common in the major ranges of Arizona, Utah, New Mexico, Colorado, and northward. It is even more common in the northern Rockies and the rest of the coastal states.

COLLECTING: The roots and basal leaves in the fall, dried loosely on newspapers, or Method C.

MEDICINAL USE: The crushed leaves and roots are soothing and mucilaginous like those of many other orchids and may be used fresh in the same manner as true Plantain, i.e., for scratches, inflammations, insect bites, and such. Several crushed leaves, washed well and steeped in clean water, makes a soothing eyewash for first aid. The whole plant can be dried, roots and leaves, and ground into a powder with a grain mill or blender. This is used in the same manner as slippery elm, comfrey root, taro, lotus root, kudzu, or clay, that is, as a drawing poultice.

RED CLOVER

Trifolium pratense   Leguminaceae

APPEARANCE: This is a substantial clover, larger than our other true clovers, with a height anywhere from one to three feet. It is perennial, with many leafy branches and three-parted leaves, each one bearing a distinctive light V-shaped marking. There are two stipules or leaflets at the juncture of each branch, and all parts of the plant except the actual flowers are finely hairy. The flower heads are large and

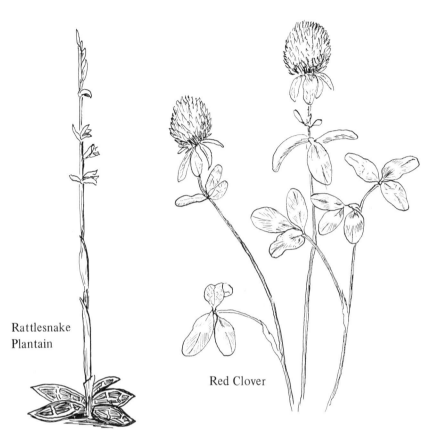

Rattlesnake Plantain

Red Clover

round, often an inch across, set inside two or three leaves that form a crude calyx. The colors of the flower heads range from pale pink to reddish purple, the center blossoms and then the edges fading into rust red as they die.

HABITAT: Erratic in California, most reliably in meadows 6,000 feet or higher where there is or has been cattle or horse pasturing. In Arizona and New Mexico they are found most frequently above 7,000 feet or in rural areas where there is plenty of moisture with mixed farming and livestock . . . and the fertilizer from same. From Colorado and Utah northwards, Red Clover can be expected anywhere.

COLLECTING: The tops, upper leaves, and blossoms, Method C. Turn them frequently as they dry; otherwise, they are prone to discoloration from fermentation or mold.

MEDICINAL USE: Red Clover is a good tasting herb tea, mainly valuable for its mineral content but also possessing mild alterative properties as well as a mild sedative effect which is useful for children and sometimes even adults. A gentle expectorant and antitussive, its value as a medicine lies in its mildness and good taste, making it one of the best maintenance liquids for the duration of any infection and, if tolerated, a tea for people with such debilitating illnesses as hepatitis and mononucleosis.

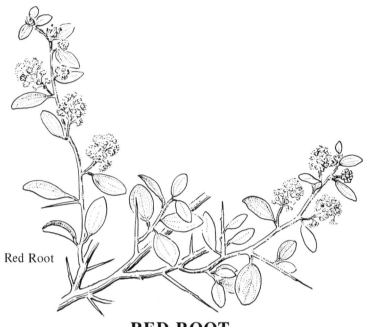

Red Root

RED ROOT

Ceanothus spp.   Rhamnaceae

OTHER NAMES: Buckbrush, Mountain Lilac, (New) Jersey Tea, California Lilac

APPEARANCE: Although a widely varied genera, several characteristics are universal. The small seed pods resemble a horned acorn, distinctly three lobed and tending to be darkly shaded where they face the sun, as if spray painted from that angle. The small delicate flowers are born on showy little puffs at the end of the straight stems that tend to stand out from the branches at sharp, almost right angles. In California, particularly along the coast, there are several attractive species that grow as small trees with beautiful lilac, pink, and purple flowers; the more common types have white or cream-colored flowers, small dark green or olive-colored leaves and sparsely leaved or leafless branchlets that double as blunt "thorns." *C. cuneatus, C. greggii,* and *C. fendleri* are the primary species of this type, the first two appearing as small shrubs from two to five feet in height, the latter from a scruffy ground cover to a small shrublet up to three feet tall. The little five-pointed lacy flowers form fragrant clusters at the ends of the branches and if rubbed in water will form a soapy foam.

HABITAT: Widespread in all the middle mountains of our area, and in fact can be found in nearly all altitudes, from the California coastal ranges to the Mohave and Colorado deserts to 9,500 feet in the Rockies. Wherever found, if the root bark and inner pith of the hard roots has a reddish purple or brown red color it is usable.

COLLECTING: Roots in the late fall when their color is darkest, or in early spring before flowering; at any time, however, they will have some value. The plants are tough and wiry, the roots doubly so. Sharp, stout clippers or wire cutters should be used to split the roots while they are still fresh; after drying, a jackhammer may be necessary. Method C or dried in a paper bag.

MEDICINAL USE: A lymphatic remedy, stimulating lymph and intertissue fluid circulation. For tonsil inflammations, sore throats, enlarged lymph nodes, and for shrinking nonfibrous cysts. For adults, two tablespoons of the root should be boiled for twenty minutes in a quart of water and refrigerated, a third of the quart drunk an hour before each meal. A few days of this regimen will generally reduce an enlarged spleen. For those that use oriental diagnostic methods, a rounded tablespoon of Red Root and a scant tablespoon of Vervain brewed similarly and drunk for several days will help clear the meridians of the torso, pelvis, and legs. If these are longstanding blockages and the meridians either over- or undersensitive, this treatment will help to clarify diagnosis and subsequent therapy, be it acupuncture, reflexology, chiropractice, or whatever.

It is an excellent home remedy for menstrual hemorrhage, nosebleeds, bleeding piles, hemorrhoids, and old ulcers, as well as capillary ruptures from vomiting or coughing. The active substances in Red Root are ceanothic (emmolic) acid, succinic acid, oxalic acid, malonic acid, malic acid, orthophosphoric acid, and pyrophosphoric acid . . . and tannin. The tincture of California Lilac was used by Boericke for sore throat, inflamed tonsils, sinus inflammations, and diphtheria, both internally and as a gargle. The tea was formerly used as a hair tonic.

CULTIVATION: Red Root covers so many forms, variations, and species, many endemic, that cultivation is probably best with a species already growing in your same general area. It is impractical to transplant the fibrous taproot—such roots do not move well. Planting from the seeds, sewn in the fall under conditions similar to those found in the wild, is most practical. With gentle pruning, a handsome group of plants.

ROSE

Rosa spp.   Rosaceae

APPEARANCE AND HABITAT: A description of the Wild Rose seems almost superfluous. All of our wild species have a single row of petals, usually five, with many typical yellow stamens, and are distinctly smaller than cultivated hybrids. Like all basic Roses, they are pink. The stems are variously thorny and slightly waxy-sticky, the leaves rose-pinnate with five to nine leaflets. Variations of leaf numbers, petal numbers, and color, and even the presence or absence of thorniness, is common within the same species. The flowers mature into hips, the little fruit that turns from green yellow to opaque orange and finally (with a good frost) to translucent dark red. Roses are found at all altitudes in our area, but most frequently are in mountainous areas, from foothill streamsides to moist meadows above 10,000 feet. They may form thickets of two- and three-foot-tall plants or clusters of large bushes, depending on the species and growing conditions. Cultivated Roses may be used in the same manner, although the hips are mealy and rather useless unless grown in a climate that has a distinct winter season.

COLLECTING: The flowers and buds, spring to early summer, Method C. The hips after a strong frost, through to the next spring, also Method C.

MEDICINAL USE: A good treatment for diarrhea; five to ten flowers or buds steeped in hot water for twenty minutes and drunk as often as needed, generally every two or three hours, beginning at least twelve hours after the onset. Since most diarrhea serves a useful defense purpose in the body, a sensible time should be allowed for the condition to run a functional course before taking medication or an herbal remedy. Rose buds are also one of the safest and most widely used eyewashes, acting as a mild astringent, giving tone to the tissues, and shrinking capillary inflammation and redness. Two or three flowers, steeped in a half cup of water until it reaches body temperature and then strained well, is sufficient. Eyewashes generally have little substantial effect on an infection and are best suited for simple inflammation; a pharmaceutical preparation of Rosebuds is marketed by at least one company for eye use, and the flowers have been used for centuries in folk medicine.

SAGE

Salvia spp.   Labiateae

OTHER NAMES: Black Sage, Scarlet Sage, Texas Sage, Crimson Sage, Purple Sage, Hummingbird Sage, White Sage, Thistle Sage, Blue Sage, ad nauseum

APPEARANCE: First things first. This member of the mint family has square stems and opposing leaves with flowers forming (usually) substantial terminal puffs like Horehound. Many people confuse true Sage with several of the Wormwoods, such as Sagebrush, Rocky Mountain Sage, and Silver Sage. These are completely unrelated plants with alternate, usually dissected leaves; they form little balls of flowers along one or both sides of thin terminal stems. The leaves of the *Salvias* are usually rounder. These Wormwood "Sages" with their often gray color and sagey smell result in much confusion; they are, however, intensely bitter whereas the Sages are just as aromatic as a rule but usually have little bitterness. What we are dealing with here are the various wild relatives of Cooking Sage *(Salvia officinalis* and such), the kind you grow in an herb garden and use for turkey stuffing and sausage. If you use the Wormwoods as "Sage," you are guaranteed to ruin even the biggest, oldest, gamiest tom turkey you can catch, let alone the indeterminate turkoid fowls of the supermarket. Although some of the wild Sages might taste a little peculiar in stuffing, they still would be recognizable Sages.

In appearance, the plants will vary from a small, medicinally weak annual in the Rockies with no particular aroma to the strongly scented and prolific Sages of southern California, large bushes with foliage that varies from smooth silvery white to wrinkled gray green to dark shiny-sticky green. The flowers range in color from pink to red, blue, purple, and even white. The varieties of Sage are so many in the West that a local flower guide is preferable to a long discourse here. One rule of thumb with this varied family: if they are at least moderately smelly, they are useful as a remedy.

HABITAT: From the surf to the western borders of the Mohave, the Sages *own* the lower mountains of southern California, and often form pure stands of several mixed species. There are many varieties in and around the Mohave and Colorado deserts, with decreasingly useful and less common species in the rest of our area. The best sage of Arizona and New Mexico is the Texas Sage, a thick-leaved little bush with crimson flowers that frequents dry mountainsides and foothills in the southern mountains, having crinkly heart-shaped leaves, bright but small flower clusters, and a height not much over a foot and a half. The occasional *Salvias* found in the Rockies, Utah, and Idaho are atypical, feeble remedies.

COLLECTING: Method A.

MEDICINAL USE: Above all else, Sage tea will decrease secretions, from sweating, salivation, and milk secretions to mucous secretions of the sinuses, throat, and

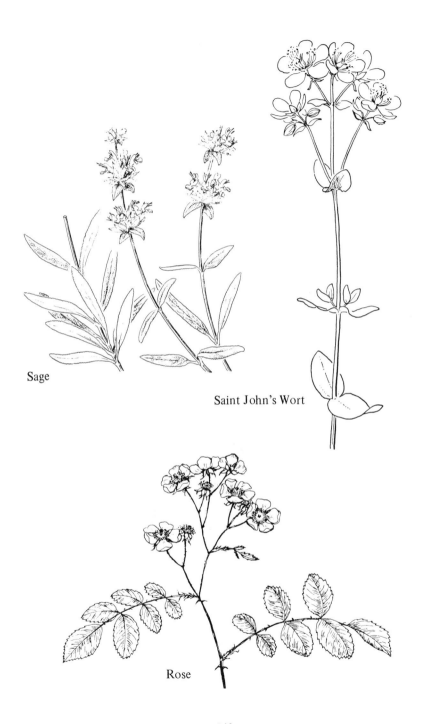

Sage

Saint John's Wort

Rose

lungs. It is the best herbal treatment for decreasing lactation during weaning in either animals or humans, a cup before each meal as long as needed. A cold cup of the tea is a good stomach tonic, particularly for ulcers and stomach inflammations. It has a substantial effect on diarrhea that is small intestinal in origin. The lukewarm tea is sufficiently bacteriostatic and astringent to make it useful for treating nearly all sore throats, both gargled and then drunk. Because it decreases sweating it is most useful alone rather than combined with such sweat stimulants as peppermint, Elder, or Yarrow. A rounded teaspoon of the crushed leaves is a reliable uterine hemostatic tea, good for heavy menstruation but inadvisable for the new mother who plans to nurse.

SAINT JOHN'S WORT

Hypericum formosum   Hypericaceae

OTHER NAMES: Hypericum, Klamath Weed *(H. perforatum)*, *H. scouleri*

APPEARANCE: This is our primary native *Hypericum*, and is a mountain dweller, unlike the widely naturalized nuisance, Klamath Weed, which is only found sparingly in our area. Our species is a delicate little perennial seldom over two feet tall, which seldom branches except to accommodate more of the terminal yellow flowers. These have five distinct petals with three clusters of numerous roselike stamens. There is often a reddish tinge to new flowers or buds. The leaves are oval to round, clasp the stems in pairs, and may have a bluish glaucous tint. The petals, sepals, and leaf margins have tiny translucent-black dots; the seed capsules are three sectioned and horned.

HABITAT: In California, both *H. formosum* and *H. anagalloides* are found in some abundance. The latter species, so named for its similarity in foliage to Scarlet Pimpernel *(Anagallis arvensis)* is a smaller plant that forms dense mats in wet sumps and spring mouths. In Arizona, New Mexico, Colorado, and elsewhere in our range, *H. formosum* is a plant of the main forest, from 6,000 to 10,000 feet, found in wet meadows, streamside flats, and semiswampy areas. The higher it grows, the more the flowers take on a butterscotch or orange color. Widespread, common, but not predictable. Difficult to identify unless in bloom. Unlike their ubiquitous relative from Europe, Klamath Weed, these two species are not particularly fond of people and are found in relatively virgin forests.

COLLECTING: Method A.

MEDICINAL USE: St. John's Wort is a useful expectorant, in doses of a teaspoon in a cup. For some it is a useful sedative or antispasmodic, while others experience little or nothing. The most effective preparations are made from the fresh plant. For a steeped oil, the finely chopped plant should be puréed in a blender with an equal volume of vegetable oil, set aside for a month or two, and then strained; this makes an excellent ointment for virtually any skin inflammations. To preserve from rancidity, a tablespoon of Compound Tincture of Benzoin or gum benzoin per pint should be added when first mixed. Hypericin, a complex substance found in the pigment of the leaf and flower dots, is used in Europe as an antidepressant. If a juicer is available, the whole fresh plant should be used, with a scant teaspoon of baking soda added to each eight ounces of liquid. The mixture should be set aside in a refrigerator overnight, an equal volume of vodka added the following morning. Without a juicer, the plant should be puréed in a blender or food processor, a teaspoon of baking soda per cup added, all allowed to steep overnight, with an equal volume of vodka added the next morning. This must age for a week and then be strained or expressed through a cloth. The reddish color that predominates in the fresh tincture (sometimes only with age) is the hypericin. Dosage varies, but is somewhere between twenty drops and a teaspoon, depending on the strength of the plant and personal metabolism. This is a perfect remedy for the "blues," sadness, irritability, insomnia, and the general grouchies. There is a slight possibility of allergylike skin eruptions in blond, blue-eyed individuals if used constantly, but I personally know of no such cases.

SELF HEAL

Prunella vulgaris   Labiateae

OTHER NAMES: Heal All, All Heal, Woundwort

APPEARANCE: A small, insignificant member of the mint family, found world-wide. It ranges in size from four inches to a foot in height, with long oval leaves, mostly basal, a few pairs along the flowering stems. The flowers are bright lavender pink, extending out of involuted layers of calyx often tinged with brown. Creeping rootstocks are the primary form of propagation, and whole clusters of little plants, both flowering and basal, can abound on one section. Although Self Heal can grow to a height of three feet, it rarely exceeds a foot in the West.

HABITAT: Streams, runoff, and very moist shady places in our area. Not a prolific plant, it is nonetheless thoroughly dispersed, generally from 3,000 to 10,000 feet, from the Santa Monica Mountains to the coastal ranges of Santa Cruz, to Flagstaff, the Cochise Stronghold, the Gila Wilderness, Medicine Bow, and the mountains above Santa Fe, i.e., a little almost everywhere. If you see one plant (usually by luck), you will probably find several hundred along the stream or meadow; in fact, you have probably stepped on a dozen before seeing the first. A secretive little plant.

COLLECTING: Does not fit the usual methods. Since the bulk of the plant is around the base, clip just above the root and bundle below the flowers. Dry in the usual manner. For juicing, place the fresh plants in a plastic bag, seal, and keep in shade until used; rinse well in cold water immediately before juicing.

MEDICINAL USE: Although probably not worth scouring marsh and muck to find because of any profound curative value, if you find it, pick it, for it is a pleasant, genial remedy, tasty, and useful for mild fevers, gum inflammations, and sore throats. The fresh plant, as its various names might signify, is a soothing poultice for bruises and scrapes. The moistened leaves can be applied to eyelids and forehead when they're hot and tired, and the crushed leaves and flower spikes are astringent and anti-inflammatory for bites and scratches. The fresh juice, preserved with twenty-five percent vodka or ten percent alcohol, can be used as a vulnerary, relatively ouchless, for treating childhood wounds. The dried plant in tea makes a good gargle for sore gums and throat, upset stomach, mild dysentery, and excess menstruation.

CULTIVATION: Self Heal makes a good, self-seeding ground cover in very moist areas of a garden that are also fairly shady. Seeds are difficult, so use root cuttings in the spring placed one-half inch below the soil and mudded up every few days until sprouted.

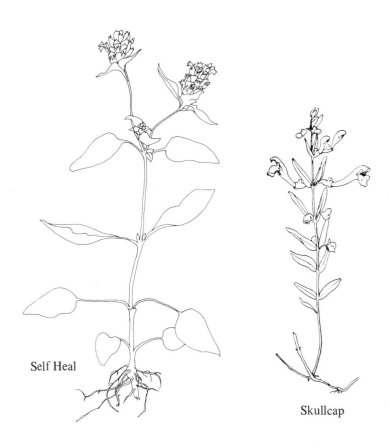

Self Heal

Skullcap

SKULLCAP

Scutelleria spp.   Labiateae

APPEARANCE AND HABITAT: One species, *S. laterifolia,* is a migrant from the eastern states and is quite different from those native to the West. It is usually found with running water, often in association with Bugleweed and the true mints, Poleo and Spearmint. It is smaller but similar in appearance; when one plant is found along a creek, many more are probably right in the same area, partially hidden by larger plants. It is a member of the mint family, and has the usual square stems and opposite leaves; when not blooming it takes a sharp eye to tell Skullcap from the surrounding mints. The flowers, in this species only, grow on little stems branching from the axils of the upper leaves, and virtually bisect the right angles formed by the leaves and stem. The flowers are small and bright blue, the whole floral stem between one and two inches long. This species may also be confused with the water-dwelling speedwells, plants that also bear small blue flowers on upper axillary stems. Speedwell, however, has competely round stems, with a bland, green taste, whereas all of the Skullcaps are more or less bitter, with a pronounced four-sided stem.

Our native Skullcaps are quite distinctive from this species, especially when in flower; like it, however, they are nondescript when not flowering. The blooms, solitary or opposite paired, are generally blue or purple. They extend out well beyond the leaves, having a long tubular body with distinctly two-lipped corollas, the upper hooded, the lower apronlike and outward-downward. The name Skullcap comes from the resemblance of the flowers to a hat (although some sources relate this to the peculiar fruit capsules). The blossoms have always reminded me of a group of malevolent little birds screeching for food. The native species are found in moist rock crevices, meadow edges, and gravelly hillsides, sporadically distributed from 2,000 to almost 10,000 feet. Not to be looked for, they are stumbled upon, in bloom from late spring to midsummer. Fortunately, when they are encountered they will be abundant in that particular area and, being perennials with durable roots, will grow back after cutting. As they are seldom taller than eighteen inches, actively searching for Skullcap can be maddening. A trip to your nearest herbarium for locality is wise.

COLLECTING: Method A, or, if possible, a fresh plant tincture. The roots may be collected for the same uses but their use is not advisable during pregnancy as they possess some steroidlike functions of an indeterminate nature not found in the foliage.

MEDICINAL USE: A sure treatment for almost any nervous system malfunction of a mild or chronic nature, from insomnia to fear to nervous or sick headaches, and as a basic palliative-restorative when pasturing-out from stress. It has been used in weaning individuals from barbiturate addiction as well as in lessening withdrawals from Valium and meprobamate abuse, avoiding some of the latter-stage convulsions and frenzies. In combination with *white* (uncured) oriental or American ginseng, it is very effective in treating the d.t.'s of alcoholism; a total of one-half ounce of Skullcap, one-fourth ounce of ginseng each day, small frequent doses preferable. Otherwise, an average dose is a scant to rounded teaspoon, *boiled* slowly for thirty minutes and drunk as needed. The tincture should be made from the fresh plant if possible, and may be taken in doses ranging from five to thirty drops or more. In treating chronic nervous system or stress problems with Skullcap it is almost essential to completely cease sucrose (refined sugar) intake, weaning from the sugar habit with dried or juiced fruits and increasing whole food carbohydrate intake.

More specifically, it can be used in treating the motor symptoms of Sydenham's (Rheumatic) Chorea, and will sometimes allay some of the pain in the earlier stages of Multiple Sclerosis. Best when the fresh tincture is used, usually in small five- to ten-drop doses, but a scant teaspoon of the dried herb may also suffice. An adventurous physician could try gradually supplanting diphenylhydantoin (Dilantin) with a fresh tincture or tea in cases of idiopathic epilepsy without demonstrable lesions, particularly when therapy has been based on a single childhood seizure or there have been obvious improvements in EEG readings. This would probably not be of much help when previous therapy has combined Dilantin and barbiturates.

SPEARMINT

Mentha spicata (viridis)   Labiateae

OTHER NAMES: Yerba Buena

APPEARANCE: *The* mint. The most common cultivated and the most common wild mint, a description is almost unnecessary. The leaves, which grow in pairs on square stems, are round, finely toothed, and distinctly wrinkled. The stems reach an average height of two feet, are bright green, and are topped in late summer by spikes of lavender or purple flowers. All parts of the plant have the friendly Spearmint smell. Curled mint *(M. crispa)* and apple mint *(M. rotundifolia)* are often encountered, both with similar scents. All mints in the West except Poleo *(M. arvensis)* are garden escapees, native originally to Europe or Asia. Such being the case, and a dozen or so hybrids having also gone feral, the resultant mix can be called "Spearmint," as they have crossbred without consideration of taxonomy and have retained the basic smell. Much like purebred cats mating and eventually becoming tabbies again. Two distinctive mints are occasionally encountered, but neither is found in abundance. Peppermint *(M. piperita)* is distinguished by smaller leaves and a sharper, less sweet odor; lemon mint *(M. citrata)* is found in a few streams in the California coastal ranges, distinguished by its candied citron scent, strong, thick, purplish stems, and bright purple terminal flower puffs.

HABITAT: Wet places throughout our range, from streamside to the lips of embankments. Usually found in stands, the creeping roots filling in all possible growing area. Generally single stalked above ground, branching plants can be found in the drier periphery of stands.

COLLECTING: Method A. Make sure the bundles are bone dry before stripping off the leaves.

MEDICINAL USE: Menthol, the most active of the mint-derived substances, is found in only small quantities in Spearmint, the primary active ingredient being carvone, a substance also found in dill and caraway seeds. The main value of Spearmint is its almost complete lack of toxicity and the ability of even the sickest person to tolerate the tea. It is its very feebleness that makes it so useful. Soothing to the stomach and a mild diuretic and diaphoretic, it has mild vasodilating characteristics, imparting a pleasant warm glow to the drinker. Along with vanilla, Spearmint is a universally enjoyed scent. In traditional New Mexican and Hispanic usage, Yerba Buena (Spearmint) is the only liquid given to a birthing mother, considered helpful as a mild uterine astringent and aiding in postpartum contractions. In California, Yerba Buena is applied to a little vine mint *(Satureja chamissonis)* that frequents wet, shady areas, and can be used for the same purposes.

CULTIVATION: Planting around a dripping faucet is always safe; otherwise, moist, fairly rich ground and a fair amount of shade. Does well along north and south sides of buildings. The seeds are nearly useless; get a root cutting from a friend or the nearest stream. It can be started in water and transplanted after rooting, or shoved under some mud and watered frequently until it sprouts. Very hardy, once established.

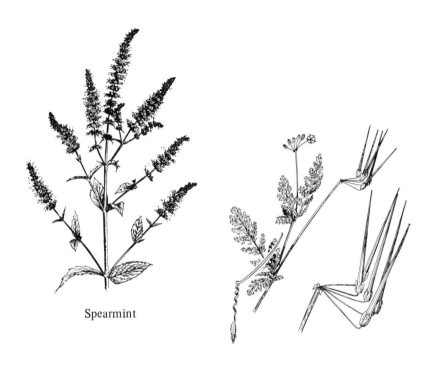

Spearmint

Storksbill

STORKSBILL

Erodium cicutarium   Geraniaceae

OTHER NAMES: Filaree, Alfilerillo, Heron's Bill

APPEARANCE AND HABITAT: A cosmopolitan weed, found throughout the world, but probably introduced originally into the Southwest by the Spanish. The name refers to the long, pointed seeds that resemble a needle or a long beak. Actually five seeds bound into one column, they separate gradually into corkscrews that straighten when wet and recoil when dry, having the effect of driving themselves into the ground. When they're green, little children put them together and play "scissors." The flowers are tiny and pink to red, resembling their relative the geranium. The plant, an annual, begins as a dense basal rosette of finely divided, delicate leaves, the flowering stalks either short or long, with many flowers and seeds, green or died back, interspersed in a weedy, straggly mass. The plant blooms as early as possible and until frost or drought has killed it, surviving several years in southern California coastal dunes or three months in alpine meadows. Highly adaptable, both in growing conditions and size, it may never exceed the diameter of a thumbnail along a dry road but may become two feet or more in diameter in rich meadows. Storksbill has a single turnip-like taproot.

149

COLLECTING: The whole plant, root and all, when just flowering, usually in mid or late spring. It can be bound by the tap roots and dried, or use Method C.

MEDICINAL USE: A mild uterine hemostatic and a diuretic for water retention, rheumatism, or gout. Not a potent plant, a fair amount is needed for effect depending on the use. Storksbill is a traditional afterbirth remedy in northern Mexico and New Mexico, said to reliably decrease bleeding and help prevent infection. A tablespoon of the root and leaves are brewed into tea and drunk three or four times a day. A tablespoon of the plant with an equal part of comfrey leaves or borage steeped in a pint of water and used for douching is considered a reliable treatment for cervicitis, especially if it has been preceded by vaginal inflammation and no uterine infection is involved. For joint inflammations a fair amount of the tea is consumed and the wet leaves used for a poultice for several days, the swellings subsiding by the third or fourth day. Chronic use of diuretics is inadvisable, of course, but Storksbill has little adverse effect on the kidneys and is an older herbal treatment in China for hematuria, particularly from kidney trauma. One of many reliable herbs for heavy, painful menstruation.

OTHER USES: The plant, picked in spring before flowering, is a good pot herb or can be chopped fresh in salads.

STRAWBERRY

Fragaria spp.   Rosaceae

APPEARANCE: The obvious, to those who have grown the plant: three-lobed leaves, sometimes fuzzy, sometimes almost smooth; pretty little white and yellow flowers that turn into the wild Strawberries so seldom encountered (everything in the mountains that moves gets to them first); the frequent long pink runners that leapfrog across the ground, rooting and starting new plants. In other words . . . Strawberries. Seldom found taller than eight or nine inches.

HABITAT: From 5,000 to 7,000 feet in the inland mountains of southern California (San Bernardino Mountains, etc.), the Sierra Nevadas from Tular County northwards, and above 7,000 feet in the moist mountains of Arizona, New Mexico, and north. Generally above the Ponderosa belt, in wet meadows, forest clearings, and northern slopes. A plant of shady areas.

MEDICINAL USE: A mild and feeble remedy, the leaves and stems make a pleasant, slightly tart tea. Its ease of administration makes it useful where stronger herbs might be objectionable. Like Raspberry leaves, it has a mild astringent effect useful for pregnancy, convalescence, and chronic stomach sensitivity, with a mild but noticeable diuretic effect. It has a tendency to acidify the urine and can have some value in lower urinary tract conditions associated with urine alkalinity. The tea, drunk frequently, will help hematuria and diarrhea. The same tea, especially with the rootstalks included, can be used as a douche for vaginitis and as an enema for diarrhea. The roots alone are particularly useful for obstinate dysentery; a piece of the root held against sore gums or a burst gumboil will help in shrinking the inflammation. I met a Scottish gentleman on one occasion who placed the fresh leaves under his dentures whenever his gums were inflamed and sore.

CULTIVATION: The plant likes slightly acid, rich soil, with plenty of moisture and shade. Easily transplanted from freshly rooted runners and sufficient native soil to hold the thread-roots intact.

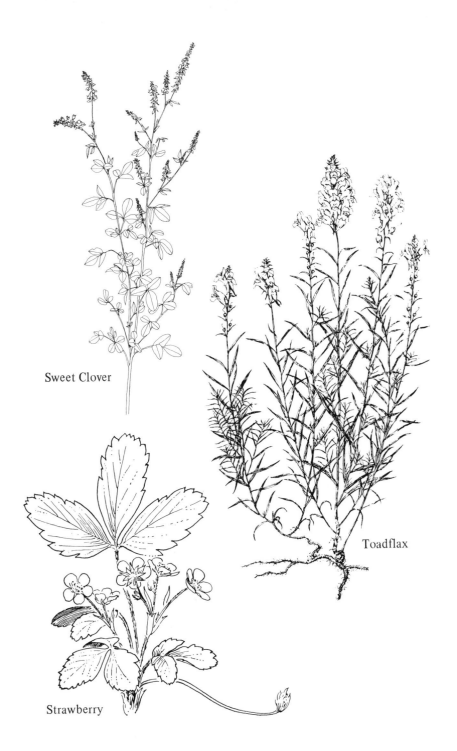

Sweet Clover

Toadflax

Strawberry

SWEET CLOVER

Melilotus officinalis, M. alba　　Leguminosae

OTHER NAMES: Melilot, Yellow Sweet Clover, White Sweet Clover, Alfalfón

APPEARANCE: A typical three-leaved clover growing from two to five feet in height, sometimes larger in stream beds. Resembling Alfalfa (and indistinguishable from it prior to blooming), the Sweet Clovers tend to grow taller and stemmier during the summer, with less leaf and more stem, eventually making a very scraggly autumn weed with little round barbed seeds that cling to the clothes of the autumn hiker. Unlike the smaller clovers and Alfalfa, the flowers of Yellow and White Sweet Clover are found in little spikes; they have a feeble but distinctive scent reminiscent of violet and vanilla. The plants flower from early summer to the first snows of November.

HABITAT: A people plant, miles upon miles of mountain roadsides are often covered with the plants, the yellow variety generally in blossom before the white and slightly smaller. Both plants may be found growing side by side. If established in streams, the plants can cover whole basins and flood plains as well as streamsides, the area becoming as impassable as Willow thickets.

COLLECTING: Method A; best to pick when first flowering, when there are a greater proportion of leaves to stems. The stems become rather tough when dry, so the fewer the better. Only the dry plant is used.

MEDICINAL USE: Sweet Clover is a traditional external poultice for sore breasts and mild mastitis, as well as any other soft tissue inflammation. The tea has been used in many countries as a stomach soother and for chronic flatulence, particularly following intestinal infections. The tea has a pleasant vanilla flavor and can be drunk simply for its taste. The vanilla scent so evident upon drying results from the presence of coumarin, a substance also found in sweet vernal grass (zubrowka), woodruff, tonka beans, tarragon, and freshly cut Alfalfa. The leaves can be used instead of woodruff for making May wine (commercial woodruff is seldom fresh enough) and can be steeped in vodka to approximate zubrowka nastoika, the traditional sweet vodka of Poland and western Russia. The dried bundles have a pleasant, light effect and tend to alleviate the depression of convalescence when they are hung about and allowed to scent the air. Many a sodbuster in the last century warded off the dirt and mold smell of early spring in a dirt cabin with bundles of Sweet Clover picked the previous summer.

Care should be taken with any long-term use of the tea. Coumarin can combine in many inappropriate ways with prescription drugs, resulting in peculiar and unpredictable compounds. One of the basic anticoagulant drugs used in present medicine, bishydroxycoumarin (Dicumarol), was discovered quite by accident when a rash of fatal internal bleeding among cattle was found to have been due to the eating of rotten Sweet Clover that had been bundled for fodder before it was dry. The fermentation within the bales of wet plants had turned the coumarin into bishydroxycoumarin.

OTHER USES: The dried leaves and flowers can be used as pillow stuffers. The leaves have been used in the manufacturing of cheese such as Gruyère and Schabzieger, and also make a pleasant adjunct to pipe tobacco or as an aromatic addition to herbal smoking mixtures.

TOADFLAX (see color plate)

Linaria vulgaris   Scrophularaceae

OTHER NAMES: Butter-and-Eggs, Wild Snapdragon

APPEARANCE AND HABITAT: This is a small, wild snapdragon with thin, almost grasslike leaves crowded along a round, smooth stem and bearing a terminal showy panicle of yellow and orange flowers. Toadflax usually forms moderate to large stands of individuals, frequently found growing down (or up) moderate slopes and along canyon bottoms and stream embankments. The average plant is around eighteen inches, but in sheltered or favorable locations some will be three feet or taller. Not overly common in California, it is found in abundance in the mountains of the rest of the West, from 6,000 to 11,000 feet, and is frequent around mountain resorts and towns. An introduced plant, it likes moisture as well as a moderate amount of sun, is adaptable to many circumstances, and has erratic dispersal in our area; in some forests almost a dominant plant, rare in other areas. Dalmatian Toadflax *(L. dalmatica),* another introduced garden plant, is abundant here and there. It has the same snapdragon yellow and orange flowers, but is taller, thicker stemmed, and the leaves, thick and profuse, clasp the stems with broad bases. It has identical uses.

COLLECTING: The flowering stems, Method A.

MEDICINAL USE: A strong, sure, but potentially irritating liver stimulant. It is generally used in combination with other herbs for a liver tonic, cleanser, or "flush." A scant teaspoon is a reasonable amount to consume at one time, along with such herbs as Burdock, Dandelion, Yellow Dock, or Red Root. It is perhaps our best native hepatic remedy for chronic liver inflammations and hepatitis flare-ups; a rounded teaspoon in tea several times a day can quickly reduce bilirubin levels towards normal. Those who have not had liver problems may find it of little subjective value; this can be due as much to their inability to recognize the feelings of an overworked liver as anything else. Those who have contracted hepatitis retain a strong memory of their peculiar symptoms, tiredness, ennui . . . even a specific taste . . . and can relate to such symptoms quickly. The rest of us may just crawl weakly out of bed for a few mornings and not be aware of the cause. Toadflax seems to have little effect on normal levels of bile production but will stimulate its secretion when insufficient.

CULTIVATION: An attractive little plant for cultivation, the seeds should be sown in well drained, moderately mulched soil in the fall. Flourishes better where frosts are pronounced.

TOBACCO

Nicotiana glauca, Nicotiana attenuata   Solanaceae

OTHER NAMES: Wild Tobacco, Punche, Coyote Tobacco, Tree Tobacco, Indian Tobacco, "Mustard Tree"

APPEARANCE: The only perennial Tobacco in our area is *N. glauca* or Tree Tobacco, a plant naturalized from Peru and apparently first introduced from a botanical garden in Los Angeles during the last century. It is a long, scraggly bush from four to fifteen feet tall, composed of tall, unkempt branches and stems and foliage that are completely smooth and glaucous. The basal leaves, large and verdant in the spring and early summer, are oval and bluish green with long, succulent leaf stems. The flowers are a pale, sickly yellow, completely tubular until the end where they flare out slightly to form five tiny lobes. The flowers average slightly longer than an inch, with slight waist below the corolla. The seeds are small brown capsules. The smaller stem leaves are alternate, persisting all year. The native Tobaccos, *N. attenuata* the most common, are annuals, from one and a half to four feet high and covered densely with little sticky hairs; the plants often have a brownish dirty appearance from adhering dust. The leaves are also long stemmed, pronouncedly basal, the lower oval, often with clasping petioles, the upper lanceolate, sometimes reduced almost to scales. The flowers are long and tubular, white to light green, from one to two inches long, flaring out to a small, five-lobed corolla. The seed capsules are brown green, sticky, and, like all of the plant, ill smelling. Some exceptions are *N. trigonophylla* with stemless, clasping leaves, and *N. bigolovii,* having larger and showy petunialike flowers. Both are predominantly higher desert species. Except for *N. glauca,* all of our native Tobaccos present a strongly triangular silhouette, with large basal leaves and progressively shorter leaves up the usual single flowering stem.

HABITAT: Tree Tobacco is common throughout the southern coastal and inland ranges of California, from San Diego to the Hollywood Hills to Santa Cruz, eastward through the southern sections of Arizona, New Mexico, and Texas; generally in dry stream beds and arroyos in the foothills, seldom ascending above 4,000 feet, usually lower. This species has a knack for filling in the empty nooks and crannies and can be found growing in the most preposterous places. I once observed a larger plant growing virtually upside down from the eroded lip of an arroyo below a freeway in California, at least fifteen feet "high," a whole host of offspring growing from the concrete tailings in the gully below. All the plants as well as the parent were a picture of health with nary an insect bite to mar their blue green leaves. Tree Tobacco does not need much moisture but does require spring runoff and usually follows the water from high dry canyons down to sandy flood plains.

The native species are found here and there almost throughout our area, from California to west Texas and north to Colorado, Utah, and Nevada, most frequently in meadows, flats, flood plains, dry streams, and outright desert, from sea level to 7,000 feet. They are never as predictable as *N. glauca* but are always found in stands and can be encountered at almost anytime outside of city areas. I have found the native Tobaccos growing in such diverse localities as the middle of a "recreational" trailer park in the Santa Monica Mountains of California and a dead, sandy wash outside of Yuma, Arizona.

COLLECTING: Method A. (For smoking, see Other Uses.)

MEDICINAL USE: Tobacco is mainly used externally as an analgesic poultice, the plant crushed and laid between two hot, moistened cloths and applied to sore muscles, joints, sunburn, or other external pain. One-half cup of the chopped plant can be boiled with a quart of water for twenty minutes, strained, and the tea added to bath water. This will relieve the pains of such things as hemmorrhoids, menstrual cramps, and muscle bruises. A fine liniment can be made by steeping one cup of the dried plant and a tablespoon of cayenne pepper in a quart of rubbing alcohol for at least a week. *Internal* use of wild Tobacco, however, can be near disastrous.

CULTIVATION: Easily accomplished from the ripe seeds and needs no special attention beyond dirt, sun, and water.

OTHER USES: All of our Tobaccos have been used at various times for smoking, particularly in Indian ceremonies. At present, the Tree Tobacco has the widest use amongst the various tribes. The leaves contain more complex substances than the native species, ranging from anabasine to harmine, the resultant smoke having rather different effects than commercial Tobacco. The basal leaves of all our Tobaccos can be aged for smoking; raw green-dried (Method A) leaves can be disgustingly deranging. The aging results in breaking down of the leaf sugars, volatile and fixed oils, and alkaloids. The large, healthy bottom leaves should be picked in the spring, dried in the full sun or hung up loosely indoors. If the latter method, allow two or three months at least for aging; in the sun, four or five days. The dried leaves should be carefully laid out and sprayed with a fine mist of warm water until saturated and rubbery. For maximum mildness, lay them carefully along a length of muslin or cheesecloth and roll up into a light cylinder (cloth outside only), tying firmly with twine or a number of rubber bands and allowing to ferment for a month. Spray every once in awhile with water or rum or whisky, avoiding a sugared liquid, since the added sugar in the leaves of American and European Tobaccos is perhaps the most carcinogenic aspect of commercial "curing." After a month, unwrap the Tobacco and cut across with a razor blade or sharp knife to the desired consistency. Like any Tobacco, keep slightly moist after cutting. Every species has a different taste and endless variations in flavors are possible. This crude curing is recommended for the more hard-core smokers amongst you, since it will probably send a menthol pseudocigarette smoker off into the bathroom with green paroxysms. No lumberjack-macho intended; we have simply been weaned, like so many of our processed functions, from the hot, slightly offensive and acquired taste of actual Tobacco.

Tobacco has a number of uses as an insecticide, and wild Tobacco has several distinct advantages over commercial Tobacco if you wish to make your own plant spray. Uncured plants contain a far higher content of pyridine alkaloids, including nicotine, and in the case of *N. glauca,* their more effective precursor, anabasine. Further, wild Tobaccos are virtually free of tobacco mosaic virus (common in cheap Tobacco), which can infect the leaves of tomatoes, potatoes, chilis, and other related plants. For spraying aphids and other leaf suckers, steep one cup of the chopped dried (Method A) plant in a quart of boiling water for one-half hour, adding a tablespoon of baking soda or liquid detergent, turn off heat, and cool to room temperature. This tea can be sprayed with a fine mist full strength on a large vegetable garden or diluted one-half for house plants. It may stunt the flowers of a few plants, so test one first, allowing a day for any adverse effects to show themselves. The commercial equivalent is Black Leaf 40.

UVA URSI

Arctostaphylos uva-ursi   Ericaceae

OTHER NAMES: Bearberry, Kinnikinnik, Creeping Manzanita, Coralillo, Hog Cranberry

APPEARANCE: The leaves, like all Manzanitas, are leathery and plastic to the touch; the flowers are pink and flesh colored, maturing into bright red berries, mealy and rather tasteless. The plant is a mat or a trailing vine depending on where it is growing; new spring growth may attain the height of eight or ten inches. The long trailing stems run just below ground level, generally in loose, coniferous mulch. The flowers and especially the berries are found on the underside of the stems. The leaves are heart shaped or oval and strongly veined in the center, the

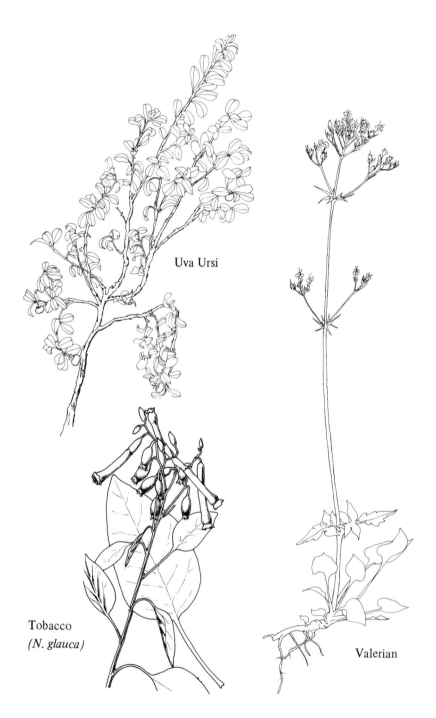

Uva Ursi

Tobacco
(N. glauca)

Valerian

edges usually somewhat concave. The bark of the stems, when washed, will show reddish dark brown with much shredding. Dead brown leaves on the underside of the trailing stems become part of the growing mulch.

HABITAT: High mountains, from 6,000 to 9,000 feet; in open clearings and new burns, forming mats here and there or trailing down over the lips of dirt roads, generally in conifers. For convenience, long trailing downhill stems are the preferable form for picking. Some strains are to be found along sandy slopes of Pacific beaches from northern California to Alaska, but in our area Uva Ursi is a mountain plant. Sporadic in most areas.

MEDICINAL USES: A specific treatment for nephritis, cystitis, and urethritis as well as an antilithic for kidney and bladder stones. The primary glycosides, arbutin and ericolin, are broken down into hydroquinone and methylhydroquinone, both disinfecting to the urinary tract. The tea can be irritating to the mucosa of the stomach in large frequent doses. It is a mild vasoconstrictor to the endometrium of the uterus and is useful for painful and heavy menstruation, although, like Manzanita, should not be used during pregnancy in any large quantity because of the possibility of decreased circulation to the fetus. The leaves make an excellent sitz bath after childbirth, helping to reduce inflammation and prevent infection. One-fourth cup of the leaves is boiled in a gallon of water for twenty minutes and cooled to body temperature, the bath taken every morning for three or four days. Uva Ursi also has value as a diuretic in cardiac-related dropsy. Highly astringent, a strong tea of the leaves makes a good wash for minor skin irritations, heat rash, hives, and thrush. Maximum effect in urinary tract usage is obtained either from tincturing (one-half teaspoon in water as needed) or by soaking the leaves in an equal volume of brandy for several days and making a tea from the wet leaves, a teaspoon for a cup.

OTHER USES: The name Kinnikinnik, often applied to Uva Ursi, derives from its frequent use alone or in mixtures as a smoking herb. The leaves are a tanning agent in Scandinavia.

CULTIVATION: From dormant roots in early spring. An excellent ground cover for hillsides and a plant that prevents erosion, it has been widely used in some areas for road and highway embankments. Very hardy in almost any weather. I have no information on starting from seeds, but it should be attempted along with root transplants.

VALERIAN

Valeriana spp.   Valerianaceae

OTHER NAMES: Tobacco Root

DESCRIPTION: A small, insignificant plant that forms little rosettes of two- or three-inch leaves in rich humus, tucked in moist crevices or attached to mossy rocks. The leaves are bright green, spade shaped, dividing into lobes as they mature, very much like mustard or cauliflower. There is one atypical species that is large and conspicuous *(Valeriana edulis)* but its medicinal effect is rather feeble. The more useful species, *V. sylvatica, V. arizonica,* and *V. acutiloba* (the first a California native, the other two found in Arizona, Nevada, Idaho, Utah, and the Rockies) are all petite. The flowers bloom in late spring and are a bright pink cluster of little mustardlike flowers with a slight but pleasant odor, atop a six- to fifteen-inch flower stalk. The basal leaves survive on into late fall and are often the last green herbs showing by the first snow. The rootstalk has a distinct and pernicious odor: when fresh, like a cross between rich dirt and Tobacco; upon drying, the precise smell of dirty socks. The little knobby roots creep along under the ground (except for *V. edulis* which has a deep yellow taproot) and have a strong brown color.

HABITAT: Moisture, above all else. If you are in the Sierra Nevadas from Tulare County north or in the major ranges of Arizona, Nevada, Utah, New Mexico, the Rocky Mountain states, you will probably find Valerian growing in moist gorges, stream embankments, and crevices. The primary prerequisites are moisture, shade, and altitude. Valerian is found from 7,000 feet and higher, although *V. arizonica* may be found as low as 5,000 feet in moist canyons in the Ponderosa belt.

COLLECTING: Roots in the fall, although in the Southwest species there are only small, joined root masses, seldom substantial in size. I personally pick the whole plants, rootlets, and leaf rosettes in the early fall, allowing the coarse mulchy dirt to fall off as they dry. Spread them out on a shady surface. If used for tincturing, purée them in a blender or juicer while still fresh and add an equal volume of brandy or vodka. Let the mush set for several weeks and strain off the solids, squeezing the remaining mash through a cloth.

MEDICINAL USES: Above all a sedative, strong and sure of effect. Useful for calming and sedating when under emotional stress or in pain. The root as a tea is very useful as an antispasmodic both for smooth and striped muscles. Valerian will lessen menstrual pain, muscle pain, bronchial spasms, and intestinal cramps, although its sedative effects may cause some befuddlement. A few individuals may find Valerian a stimulant, and indeed it does cause a short-term stimulation of circulation and respiration, but the predominant use is for sedation. The fresh root is preferable, either right out of the ground or in the form of a fresh root tincture. The activity of the fresh plant relies on two alkaloids, valerine and chatinine; upon drying, however, the Dirty Sock Factor (isovaleric acid) arises. The sedative effect is the same, but long-term ingestion of the dried root in large, chronic doses can result in melancholy and depression, very similar to bromidism. The tincture, from thirty drops to one-half teaspoon, an inch or two of the fresh root, or one-half to one teaspoon of the dried plant in tea. I personally find the taste and smell of Valerian morbidly fascinating, pleasant almost; as most people find it disgusting, the dried root may be powdered and taken in capsule form. Whole roots last almost indefinitely with their potency intact. I have seen pressed herbarium specimens of foliage with a small part of the root that were collected from the turn of the century, still stinking up the files.

VERVAIN (see color plate)

Verbena spp.   Verbenaceae

OTHER NAMES: Blue Vervain, Common Vervain, Verbana, Dormilón, Moradilla

APPEARANCE: There are three basic kinds of Vervains in the West. Type 1: Upright, hairy plants, square stemmed with widely spaced and toothed mintlike leaves. The average height is two or three feet. The plants begin as single thick-stemmed plants, branching only in midsummer or sometimes not at all, flowering in many long blue or purple spikes, the active blooms forming a ring of blossoms that appear to move up the spike as the season progresses, with seed pods

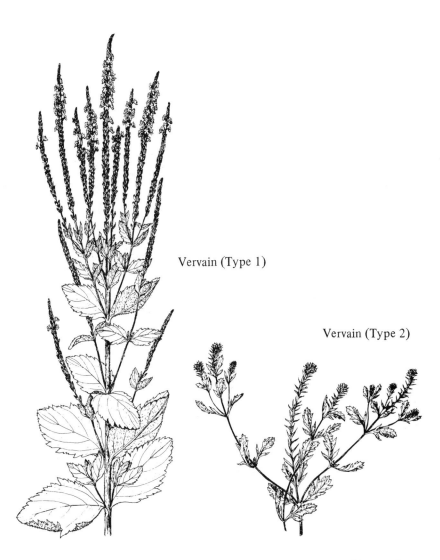

Vervain (Type 1)

Vervain (Type 2)

below and flower buds above. The toothed leaves may reach lengths of three or four inches in favored locations. Species of this type are *V. hastata, V. macdougalii,* and *V. stricta.* Type 2: A many stemmed, prostrate plant radiating out from the root in a flat mat, the deeply cleft little leaves also opposite, the many stems having dense flower spikes of a terminal nature with inconspicuous blue or purple blossoms. Species of this type are *V. bracteata* and *V. prostrata.* Type 3: These plants are similar to the species of *Verbena* cultivated in gardens. They are low, somewhat spreading plants. The stems are rarely more than a foot in length, the opposite leaves hairy and deeply cleft, the terminal flowers flattened puffs of magenta or purple, occasionally pink, blooming from middle spring to fall. Small but conspicuous because of their many showy flowers. Species of this last group are *V. canadensis, V. bipinnatifida, V. ambrosifolia, V. ciliata,* and *V. wrightii.* These are botanical headaches, with many varieties, local variations, and interbreeding the rule. I was in a university herbarium one afternoon and observed a heated argument between a student and two instructors taking place over a binocular microscope. Each person had a different and vocal identification for the poor little purple flower head under the lenses. Its nomenclature in Moore's Simplified Nonbotanical Classification System (MSNBCS) would have been *Verbena* Type 3 . . . but no one was asking.

HABITAT: Type 1 is generally a mountain plant, *V. macdougalii* most common in Arizona and the southern Rockies, the others common to California, from 2,500 feet in the coastal mountains to 5,500–8,500 feet eastward. The decumbent Type 2 Vervains are found at all altitudes, generally in waste places and dry foothill flats. Type 3 can be found from Barstow eastward in California (2,000–5,000 feet) and is in great abundance in the drier mountains and mesas of Arizona, Utah, Colorado, New Mexico, Texas, Nevada, etc.

COLLECTING: Method A while in flower, preferably July or August. In upright species only the leaves and flowers are saved, the thick lower stems discarded. The smaller types are used totally; stems, leaves, flowers, even roots. Because of the hairiness of the Vervains, all should be washed before hanging.

MEDICINAL USE: Vervain is broadly active medicinally, serving as a sedative, diaphoretic, diuretic, bitter tonic, and antispasmodic. It is one of the best palliatives for the onset of a virus cold, particularly with upper respiratory inflammation. It will promote sweating, relax and soothe, allay feverishness, settle the stomach, overall producing a feeling of relaxed well-being. It is especially useful for children who become fidgety and cranky when first feeling ill, running around in a droopy, hyperactive fashion, or for the child who has spent three hours in bed and is bored to tears but by no means well enough to play in the snow. The dose for children is one-half to one teaspoon as needed, for adults up to a tablespoon. Larger quantities of Vervain can produce nausea and vomiting and in fact it was formerly employed as an emetic. The tea is an effective sedative for insomnia and, like Hops, will settle a nervous stomach. In treating sprains and deep bruises, the tea will aid in reabsorption of blood from the ruptured tissues, two or three cups a day for at least three or four days. The tea is bitter and can be made more palatable if combined with lemon grass, lemon balm (especially good), peppermint, or wintergreen tea. The latter may counteract the diaphoretic properties of Vervain. Sweeten with honey if needed. The active principles of the Vervains are the glycoside verbenalin and tannin.

CULTIVATION: The showy varieties (Type 3) are excellent garden flowers with a long blooming season. Cultivation is from root divisions taken in the spring or seeds planted in the fall. They grow best in fairly poor sandy soil and will often self-seed and spread year after year. Some of our native Vervains are available in commercial seed packets or from nurseries. Why some gardeners grunt, wheeze, and pray over their little flowers that belong in Maine or Brittany, not Escondido, when as pretty a plant as the Type 3 Vervains would probably grow in the cracks of their sidewalks . . . well, it's beyond me.

WILLOW

Salix spp.   Salicaceae

OTHER NAMES: Black Willow, Yellow Willow, Sandbar Willow, Jara, Jarita, etc.

APPEARANCE: The taxonomy of Willows is almost past knowing; unlike their close relatives, the Poplars, Willows change, mutate, and adapt from stream to stream. This drives botanists to mild frenzies . . . or at least another master's thesis. This needn't bother us too much—suffice it to say that there are big Willow trees with yellow, gray, or blackish bark, there are small trees with wrinkled brown bark, and there are the bushy, stemmy Willows of the streams. They are all used similarly, tend to have thin, lance-shaped leaves with short stems, are smooth and hairless, and bear catkins in the spring, either before or at the beginning of the formation of leaves. The only probable confusion would arise from the narrow-leaf cottonwood (*Populus angustifolia*) or the lance-leaf cottonwood of Arizona, Utah, Wyoming, Colorado, and New Mexico (not California). Their leaf stems are longer and the catkins are drooping, whereas those of the Willows are generally upright. Willow bark is considerably easier to peel, Poplar more difficult. Even if a mistake is made, the biochemistry and remedial uses are virtually identical in the two genera.

HABITAT: Willows are water plants first and always, and particularly in the West. Since the larger portion of moist terrain in our area is mountainous, so are most of our Willows. The smaller, stemmy Willows are found along the banks of nearly every stream in the West, and the trees can be found in almost equal abundance, from nearly sea level in the coastal mountains of California to 10,000 feet or higher in our major ranges. Abundant and plentiful, impossible to avoid. If you aren't positive in the identification of the trees, particularly when they're past blooming, stick to the little plants by the stream.

COLLECTING: The bark or twigs are the plant parts collected. If the Willow is a tree, strip the bark from the newer, smooth barked branches (they are more potent); if it is a small, trunkless Willow, cut the longer, thicker, and darker barked stems, strip the leaves off, and dry the switches in bundles. They may be cut into smaller pieces after drying and the whole stem used.

MEDICINAL USE: The values of Willow lie in the glycosides salicin and populin, as well as the ever present tannin. Its uses are many, but most specifically in the reduction of inflammations of joints and membranes. Useful for headache, fevers, neuralgia, and hay fever. The glycosides are excreted in the urine as salicylic acid, salicyl alcohol, and related compounds; this renders the tea useful for urethra and bladder irritability, acting as an analgesic to those tissues. Most of our plants are not particularly potent and a fair amount of the bark or stem is needed. Up to an ounce a day can be consumed in tea if needed, although, as in any substance with the ability to alter body functions, take no more than is needed for the problem. Willow bark is a strong but benign antiseptic, and a good poultice or strong wash is made of the fresh or dried herb. For infected wounds, ulcerations, or eczema, the plant should be boiled in twice its volume of water in a covered pot for at least half an hour, some borax or boric acid added (tablespoon to a pint of water), and the tea used externally as often as necessary. One of the essential first aid plants for the wilderness buff to know about.

WORMWOOD

Artemisia spp.   Compositeae

OTHER NAMES: Mugwort, Sagebrush, "Sage," Black "Sage," Altamisa, Estafiate, etc.

APPEARANCE: This family is large, varied, and multipurpose, but several characteristics which make it fairly easy to identify are nearly universal. Plants which don't meet those criteria are usually fairly useless as remedies. The leaves tend to be noticeably hairy, either on the underside of the leaf or on both sides; usable species are strong scented when crushed, like a cross between Sage and camphor; the flowers are round or slightly tubular balls found along the extended flower stems in unleafed, generally one-sided rows. The leaves may be lance shaped but more often are deeply cleft or irregularly fingered. When blooming, sizes of the various Wormwoods vary eight to twelve inches in the little Silver Sage of Arizona and the Rockies *(A. frigida)* to two to eight feet in the California Mugwort *(A. vulgaris* and its endless subspecies).

HABITAT: A common and successful genera, Wormwood is found throughout the world. The California Mugwort can be found in moist arroyos and canyons the whole length of the Pacific states in all coastal and inland mountain ranges, and east to Nevada. Sagebrush *(A. tridentata),* can be found throughout the West, from California to Texas, typified by large dense stands of gray green scraggly bushes with tiny three-lobed leaves and coarse, gray-barked stems and trunks. Numerous species can be found along roadsides throughout the hillsides and mountains of our area, from sea level to 11,000 feet, usually from one to two feet tall and gray green.

COLLECTING: The perennial Wormwoods can be collected at nearly any time, the annuals when just into the flowering stage. Method A for drying.

MEDICINAL USES: Nearly all species are intensely bitter and strongly aromatic, making them useful either to stimulate sweating in dry fevers or for indigestion and stomach acidity. A classic stomach tonic and bitter tonic. In addition, the hot tea (rounded teaspoon to a cup of water) has a stimulating effect on uterine circulation and will help in suppressed, crampy menstruations, particularly following illness or some emotional or physical trauma. As the name signifies, Wormwood will help expel or at least inhibit roundworm and pinworm infections, the secret being constancy, with at least two cups a day for a period of a week or two. Santonin and artemisin, lactone glycosides, are found in varying quantities in nearly all of the Wormwoods, and account for their anthelmintic properties; the diaphoretic and emmenagogue characteristics derive from the thujone and phellandrene-related substances found in the aromatic oils. Although the tea is extremely bitter, I have been informed by some people that they can actually abide the taste.

OTHER USES: All the aromatic Wormwoods have been used at one time or another for sweat baths and saunas, and particularly Sagebrush. Moistened branches are thrown onto hot rocks or bricks, the victims grimly inhaling the humid vapors until nearly prostrate. Tarragon *(A. dracunculus)* and False Tarragon *(A. dracunculioides),* small, lance-leafed plants with a vanilla-sage smell, can be found on occasion. Both the Estafiate *(A. frigida)* and the Altamisa *(A. franserioides)* have been used on occasion as a spice for corn and posole but must be used with the lightest of hand . . . their bitterness can overpower easily.

CULTIVATION: From seeds sown in the fall, although few of the genera except Santolina and Mugwort would warrant active cultivation, having a rather poor appearance. The more attractive Wormwoods are available from nurseries.

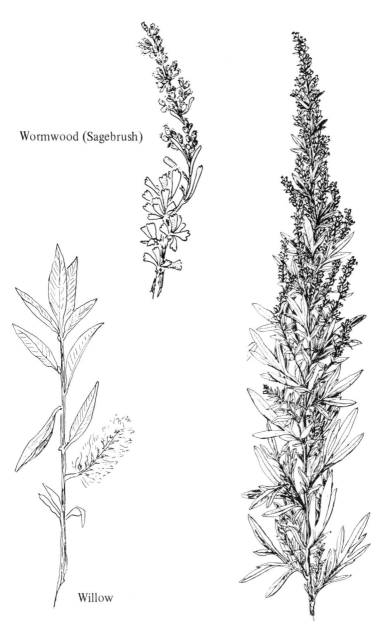

Wormwood (Sagebrush)

Willow

Wormwood (California Mugwort)

YARROW

(see color plate)

Achillea lanulosa (millefolium)   Compositeae

OTHER NAMES: Plumajillo, Milfoil

APPEARANCE: This perennial is found, in various forms, throughout the world. The leaves are fine and fernlike, forming a mat of basal leaves in spring, growing upward to the flowers in July–September. The flowers are snow white and flat topped. All parts of the plant have the typical pleasant "woodsy" scent common to the genera. Often confused with carrot and hemlock flowers, they differ markedly in scent and stem formations; carrot and hemlock flowers all spring from a single point at the end of a stem, forming an umbrellalike head, whereas Yarrow flowers start from different places along the stem, often forming several auxiliary clusters below the top. Some botanists consider the western species to be *Achillea lanulosa,* distinct from the the European species because of the downy hairs that cover the stems. Others disagree, considering them all to be the same. It is a moot question since the two types intermingle and mix without any care for nomenclature.

HABITAT: Throughout the West from Ponderosa forest to timberline and as low as 2,400 feet in the Santa Monica Mountains. Common along roads and paths, clearings, and valleys but seldom on slopes. Flowers from late May to September.

COLLECTING: The whole flowering stalk, rootlet and all. The traditional method is to gather only flowers: but the upper stems and leaves actually retain their strength longer and should be kept along with the flowers. Leaves and Flowers: Method A, or stored loosely in shopping bags until dry.

MEDICINAL USES: An effective stomach tonic, a tablespoon of the chopped plant in tea, drunk at room temperature. It has a milk laxative effect. The tea drunk hot and strong enough to be slightly bitter will stimulate sweating in dry fevers. Two or three cups a day will decrease menstruation or aid in shrinking mild hemorrhoids and colonic polyps. The fresh leaves are a reasonably effective first aid to stimulate clotting in cuts and abrasions.

OTHER USES: The dried flower stalks can be used for floral decorations and the straight naked stems, cut to about six inches in length, are used for readings in the *I Ching (Book of Changes).*

CULTIVATING: The pink and Elephant Yellow varieties are available from most nurseries. The wild Yarrow can be cultivated easily from roots with basal leaves dug in the spring.

YELLOW DOCK

Rumex crispus   Polygonaceae

OTHER NAMES: Curly Dock, Lengua de Vaca, Narrow Dock, Sour Dock

APPEARANCE: This is a common plant, found nearly world-wide. The primary characteristics of the plant are its long, curly-edged leaves, long stemmed and a foot or more in length at ground level, alternate and becoming smaller along the two- or three-foot stem, and the many clusters of three-winged flowers and seeds, green in the summer, gradually becoming a striking dark rust red in the fall. The whole plant becomes dark in color in the fall, seeds, stems, and upper leaves, and is easily distinguishable even in the snow and early spring, the brick red dead stalks covered heavily with seed panicles. The root is carrot shaped, sometimes branching, and reddish brown outside, yellow to orange inside.

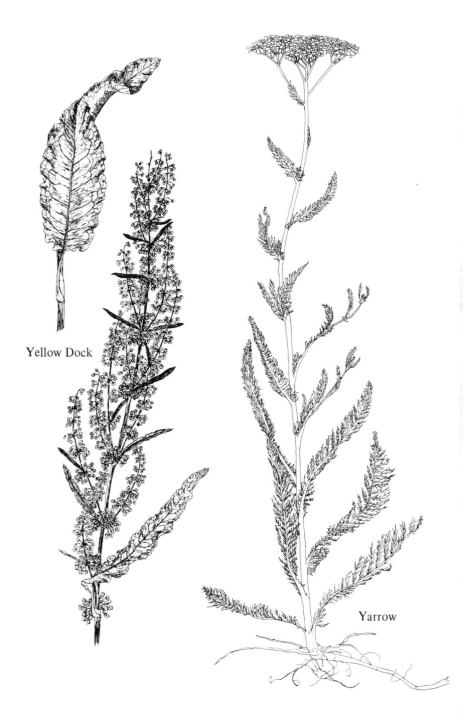

Yellow Dock

Yarrow

HABITAT: Found in all areas, it is most common in moist or formerly moist clearings, dried ditches and sumps, meadows, roadsides, and streams, from sea level to 9,000 feet and higher.

COLLECTING: Plants growing in direct water are useless, the roots light colored and many branched with large amounts of hair roots. Those plants found in drier spring meadows or along stream embankments and open areas are far preferable, usually having thick roots, dark bark, and a strong yellow or orange color inside. The darker the yellow, the stronger the root. Roots should be processed as in Method B, trimmed from the stems just below their base and the usual reddish green crown of the root, usually one-fourth to one-half inch into the crown. Always pick in the fall, the later the better, preferably in October or November.

MEDICINAL USES: The activities of Yellow Dock are due to the yellow substances chrysophanic acid and emodin, as well as variable but substantial amounts of tannin. Its primary uses are for treating constipation, blood disorders, skin diseases, rheumatism, and indigestion. For liver congestion and poor digestion of fatty foods, particularly meat and dairy products, a teaspoon of the chopped root, boiled in water, should be drunk morning and afternoon. For jaundice and post-hepatitis flare-ups, a tablespoon is boiled in water and sipped on during the day for three or four days. These quantities also have a mild but effective laxative function, and a rounded teaspoon in tea drunk before retiring for specific constipation, although not for extended use, since, as in most plant laxatives, this can result in a laxative dependence. An old remedy for skin eruptions due to internal toxicity or nervousness, one-half teaspoon in tea should be consumed at least three times a day for several days or a week. Yellow Dock is even more effective, especially when the eruptions are on oily skin of the neck and back, if combined with Burdock, sarsaparilla, and/or echinacea. The four roots together are sometimes completely effective in treating post-adolescent skin acne or eruptions related to the menstrual cycle. Drunk with or just after meals (scant teaspoon in water), Yellow Dock root will aid in reducing bleeding piles or inflamed diverticula of the colon and rectum. The root has some keratolytic activity, and is therefore useful externally for suppurating ulcers, skin infections, and poorly healed abrasions. Formerly used to slow the course of intestinal cancer, it would probably have little value combined with present cancer therapies.

CULTIVATION: This big weed is hardly graceful of demeanor and most sensible gardeners would avoid introducing it intentionally.

YERBA de la NEGRITA

Sphaeralcea coccinea, S. cuspidata   Malvaceae

OTHER NAMES: Scarlet Globemallow, Sore Eye Poppy, Yerba del Negro

APPEARANCE: The distinctive features of these two plants (and several others of the genera) are their bright little salmon, orange, or red flowers with a single stamen column in the center. The blossoms resemble little hollyhocks or hibiscus flowers, which are relatives. *S. coccinea* is a small, densely downy plant that usually grows in clumps along the ground, with many three-, five-, and seven-fingered leaves. The plants are seldom more than a few inches tall. *S. cuspidata* is considerably larger, two to four feet tall, with from one to ten stems, the leaves slightly three lobed, the center lobe far longer, the flowers clasping the upper half of the stem in a raceme. All *Sphaeralcea* are covered with tiny star-shaped hair tufts and have slimy, mucilaginous leaves when crushed or rubbed.

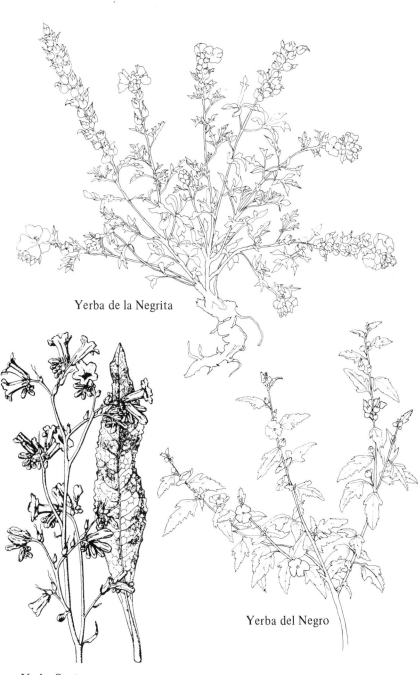

Yerba de la Negrita

Yerba del Negro

Yerba Santa

167

HABITAT: The smaller plant is found in dry plains and hills of Arizona, Utah, Colorado, New Mexico, and Texas, frequently along roadsides and vacant lots, less frequent in our more northern states. It is inconspicuous except for the flowers. The larger plant is found in all our areas. Other common species can be almost white with flowers tending towards crimson; they frequent waste places and dry slopes. Fairly adaptable to varying conditions, Yerba de la Negrita is more happened onto than looked for.

COLLECTING: Method A, in bloom.

MEDICINAL USE: A demulcent and emollient. The crushed leaves can be made into a plaster or poultice for any skin inflammation and make a soothing shoe liner for sore or blistered feet. The fresh leaves and flowers can be chewed or the dried plant brewed for tea to soothe a sore throat and hoarseness as well as minor irritability of the stomach and small intestine. A traditional New Mexican first aid for internal hemorrhoids is a little bolus of Yerba de la Negrita leaves, a pinch of *punche* (Tobacco), and saliva used as a suppository. The whole plant can be used in the same manner as marshmallow root, particularly for lower urinary tract inflammations. A cup of tea drunk three times a day until the complaint subsides; even better when combined with a few leaves of Uva Ursi, Manzanita, or Pipsissewa.

OTHER USES: A traditional hair rinse after shampooing to give body and condition the scalp. A strong tea will curl the hair if not rinsed out.

YERBA SANTA

Eriodictyon spp.   Hydrophyllaceae

OTHER NAMES: Mountain Balm, Holy Herb, Bear Plant

APPEARANCE: The official plant *(E. californica)* is not the more common of the Yerba Santas, at least in the southern half of California. In actuality, it is often difficult to tell where one species leaves off and another begins. The genera can loosely be lumped into "shiny-wooly" and "wooly-wooly" groups. To avoid corruption, botany students should not read further. Along with Yarrow and Mormon Tea, the nomenclature of the *Eriodictyon* clan is subject to almost constant revision. About the only species that avoids taxonomic miscegenation is the *E. angustifolium* of Arizona, the easternmost species in the United States. All species have greasy, pleasant smelling leaves, terminal purple or blue funnel-shaped flowers, alternate thick, slightly notched leaves, and stems with a sticky varnished surface. All Yerba Santas are bushes, between two and six feet in height. The "shiny-wooly" species are lance leaved, shiny dark green above and wooly gray yellow below. The leaves have a marked central vein and curl under along the length, becoming more pronounced upon drying. The "wooly-wooly" varieties are completely downy, more spade shaped, and have a less defined veination. In these plants, the color ranges from gray white in lower, drier areas, to bright fuzzy green at higher altitudes. The lance-leaved species are the more conspicuous, with denser foliage and a bright dark green color.

HABITAT: California coastal ranges, north to Oregon and Nevada, south to Baja California; drier slopes of the Sierra Nevadas; Arizona in the lower central mountains, from Globe, south. Elevations range from 1,000 feet in coastal ranges to 6,000 feet in inland mountains. Vast areas of northern California are covered with *E. californica,* but it is only found in the higher altitudes of southern California.

COLLECTING: Yerba Santa is strongest right after blooming, either in late spring or after a drought-breaking rain has brought out new foliage. Either bundle straight new branches, Method A, or hang larger branches singly. Pinch off the flower branches before drying.

MEDICINAL USE: An expectorant and bronchial dilator, useful in chest colds, bronchitis, asthma, and hay fever. It has mild but useful decongestant functions; all species are effective. Yerba Santa has no specific toxicities in moderate doses, and up to an ounce of the leaves can be drunk during the course of a day. For mild bronchial spasms, smoking the leaves along with the tea can improve the effects. The higher proportion of resin complex and phenols in the "shiny-wooly" varieties *(E. californica, E. parryi,* and *E. angustifolium)* makes it useful for mild bladder and urethra infections. These properties are only partially water soluble and a tincture is preferable, twenty to thirty drops in water several times a day.

OTHER USES: The disgusting taste of golden seal root can be partially masked with Yerba Santa. The fresh leaves make a tasty chewing gum, bitter and balsamic at first, with a sweet aftertaste.

CULTIVATION: From seed. Rocky, gravelly soil, well drained, with much sun, preferably on a slope. After a foot tall, drown with water twice a month and ignore otherwise. Not an easily cultivated plant.

YUCCA (see color plate)

Yucca spp.   Liliaceae

OTHER NAMES: Amole, Spanish Bayonet, Joshua Tree, Datil, Spanish Dagger

DESCRIPTION: This common and ubiquitous plant is distinct and easy to recognise. The various Yuccas have numerous spiny-tipped elongated leaves that rise in a cluster from a central stem, usually from ground level but in several species from one or more trunks. The long leaves are constantly shedding along the margins but are otherwise only armored at the leaf tips. Anyone who has backed into the aptly named Spanish Bayonet will vouch for the simple efficiency of the barbed tips, however. Often confused with Agave and beargrass, but the former has broader, thick, frequently spined leaves and a tall, obliquely branched flower stalk and the latter has much thinner, grasslike leaves that are often seen lying partially on the ground. Yucca has either a single two- to five-foot flower stalk, upright and conspicuous, or is branched like the California joshua tree with one flower stalk for each arm. The flowers are lilylike, either large and cream colored with brown flecks or smaller and yellow green. They usually open at night, closing downward in the daylight. Some of the Yucca fruit is large and succulent, particularly *Y. baccata,* but the taste tends to be mealy-bland.

HABITAT: Found most frequently in stands, often covering valleys and dry mountain slopes, it is most common in the high desert, extending up into the Juniper/Piñon belt and higher still on drier slopes in the Ponderosa belt. From nearly sea level in California to 8,000 feet on the dry sides of mountains in Utah, Arizona, New Mexico, and Colorado, throughout the West, sparse further north.

COLLECTING: The root at any time of the year. Should be split lengthwise (Method B) before drying. If for medicinal use the bark may be removed; if for washing or rinsing the hair, the bark should be left on. Use only after drying.

MEDICINAL USE: At one time considered a potential source of phytosterols, a

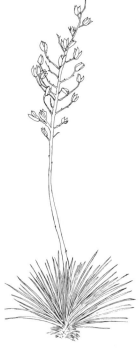

Yucca

family of plant substances used in the manufacturing of steroidal hormones, its present use is as a sudsing agent in the cosmetic and soap industries and as a home remedy for arthritic pain. Recent clinical studies have shown it to be of some use in the treatment of joint inflammations but the function is not understood. One-fourth ounce of the inner root should be boiled in a pint of water for fifteen minutes and drunk in three or four doses during the day. Arthritis being such an idiosyncratic disorder, no single treatment will help more than a percentage of people, but if Yucca tea is effective, it can relieve pain for several days afterwards. If a strong laxative effect persists, especially if accompanied by intestinal cramping, decrease the amount next time. If there are no side effects, the quantity can be increased to one-half ounce a day. Long-term daily use can slow absorption in the small intestine of fat-soluble vitamins. The tea has some value for urethra or prostate inflammations.

OTHER USES: Added to shampoo or used by itself for washing dry hair. One-half to one cup of the chopped fresh or dried root is boiled in one and one-half cups of water until suds form.

CULTIVATION: From roots dug in the late fall and replanted in well drained sandy soil.

Medicinal Plants of the Mountain West

Glossary
Therapeutic and Use Index
Plant Classifications
References and Further Reading
Index

GLOSSARY

ABORTIFACIENT: Any substance used, intentionally or otherwise, that may induce a miscarriage.

ACETYLCHOLINE: A choline ester found in many tissues of the body, most specifically the nervous system, where it facilitates the transmission of nerve impulses between nerve cells (the synapse) and between nerve endings and most muscles.

ACNE: A chronic skin problem, usually in the head and torso, manifesting itself through eruptive inflammations of the sebaceous glands and hair follicles. May be caused by steroid hormone imbalances, food allergies, dietary deficiencies (particularly Vitamin A), indigestion, stress, and faulty metabolization.

ACUTE: A type of disease having a sudden onset, severe symptoms, and a generally short duration. (Example: a head cold.) The opposite of chronic.

ADDISON'S DISEASE: A chronic deteriorative disorder of the adrenal cortex, usually of an unknown origin, characterized by a decrease in adrenalcortical function. Symptoms include increased skin pigmentation, whitish splotches, lethargy, and vomiting.

ADRENAL CORTEX: The outer covering of the adrenal glands, the two triangular endocrine glands that rest atop the kidneys. Formed in foetal development from the same tissue that becomes the gonads, the adrenal cortex secretes a number of poorly understood steroidal hormones. These regulate carbohydrate use, salt balance, reproductive functions, catabolism, and inflammation, with subtle but profound effects on every tissue of the body. Inside the cortex is the adrenal medulla, the source of adrenalin.

ADRENOCORTICAL: Of, and pertaining to, the adrenal cortex.

ALKALOID: An alkaline, nitrogen-bearing substance, usually plant derived, that reacts with acids to form a salt. Usually intensely bitter, the activity of alkaloids is such that they form a body of substances widely used in drug and herbal therapy. They generally have toxic potential. (Example: caffeine, morphine, berberine.)

ALLOPATHY: A term loosely applied by other therapies to the form of medicine practiced by physicians. More appropriately, the use of drugs or other means to antidote a disease or symptom; i.e., using aspirin to lower a fever. Since physicians can use many approaches to dealing with disease, the term only applies to a certain part of their therapeutics. The opposite of Homeopathy.

ALPINE: Those plants found predominately at and above timberline.

ALTERATIVE: A term used in galenic medicine for those plants which stimulate changes in metabolism and tissue function of a defensive nature in the presence of disease, both chronic and acute. Sometimes inaccurately used as a synonym for "blood purifiers." (Example: Elder, when used to stimulate and shorten a fever, although Elder used otherwise will not induce a fever. Its function as an alterative exists only when the body itself has begun a febrile state as a defense mechanism; without the change of metabolism called a fever, the drinking of Elder tea has no other function except as a mild diuretic.) The whole concept of alteratives is based on the premise that disease symptoms in an otherwise healthy individual are actually the external signs of internal defenses and, as such, should be stimulated and not suppressed.

ALTERNATE: A botanical term denoting an arrangement of plant organs (usually leaves) that are alternate along opposite sides of a stem, as distinct from paired or whorled.

AMINO ACID: A large group of organic, nitrogen-bearing compounds. They form the building blocks from which the body assembles, on the tissue level, the various complex proteins. Unused animo acids are excreted primarily in the urine and sweat as urea. One amino acid, also containing iodine, is the thyroid hormone, thyroxine.

ANALGESIC: A substance which relieves pain. (Example: aspirin, Poplar.)

ANESTHETIC: A substance which decreases sensitivity to pain. (Example: nitrous oxide, Oil of Cloves.)

ANODYNE: A substance which relieves pain, usually with accompanied sedation. (Example: morphine, Prickly Poppy.)

ANORECTIC (ANOREXIC): A substance (or condition) causing a decrease in appetite for food.

ANTIPYRETIC: A substance that decreases fevers. (Example: aspirin, Poplar.)

ANTISEPTIC: A substance that will prevent or retard growth of microorganisms.

ANTISPASMODIC: A substance that will relieve or prevent spasms, usually of the smooth muscles. (Example: barbiturates, Valerian.)

ANTITUSSIVE: A substance that inhibits coughing.

ARRYTHMIA: An irregularity of rhythm, usually referring to the heart.

ARTHRITIS: An inflammation of a joint, with any number of causes, usually accompanied by some alteration of joint structure.

ASTRINGENT: A substance that constricts tissues, used to stop bleeding, secretions, and the like. (Example: a styptic pencil, Oak Bark, cold.)

AXILLARY: Borne in the axil, that is, between the leaf and the stem.

BALSAMIC: Soft or hard plant or tree resins, composed of aromatic oils and acids. These are typically used as stimulating dressings and aromatic expectorants. Applied loosely to many plants that may not exude resins but have a soothing, "pitchy" scent. (Example: Balsam of Peru, Pine pitch, Yerba Santa.)

BIENNIAL: A plant that forms (generally) a basal rosette the first year of growth and a flowering stalk the second year. Most biennials die the second fall but there are many variations in cycle under different growing conditions.

BILE: A digestive and excretory secretion from the liver. Bile stored in the gall bladder is more concentrated and may be green or brown in color, whereas bile secreted directly from the liver is straw colored. Bile excretion is stimulated by the presence in the duodenum of fats, and serves as a detergent, emulsifying them and making them water soluable. Bile also serves to stimulate peristalsis in the large intestine and functions as a medium for excreting hemoglobin metabolites.

BILIARY: Pertaining to the bile secretions.

BILIRUBIN: A pigment, orange-yellow in color, that is secreted in bile as the final unusable end product of hemoglobin breakdown. It contributes to the brown color of feces and, in the case of bile duct or liver malfunctions, backs up into the blood stream to cause jaundice.

BIOFLAVONOIDS: A group of substances formerly called Vitamin P, and usually associated with ascorbic acid in natural sources. They are brightly colored and sometimes referred to as lemon or citrus bioflavonoids or simply as the "complex" part of Vitamin C Complex. They are widely used to increase the rigidity and strength of capillary walls in a number of conditions ranging from stomach ulcers to Whiskey Nose but have only marginal use in American medicine. Considering the enfeebled state of preventative medicine and preventative nutrition in this country, this is not surprising. (Example: rutin, hesperidin, citrin.)

BITTER TONIC: A substance or formula having a bitter taste and used to increase a deficient appetite, improve the acidity of stomach secretion, and slightly speed an orderly emptying of the stomach. A bitter tonic should have little if any systemic effects other than on oral and stomach functions and secretions. It usually has little effect on normal digestive functions.

BLOOD PURIFIER: A loose, somewhat simplistic name for those herbs which seem to speed up the detoxifying and excretion of waste products in the blood stream, particularly when there are resultant skin eruptions. This may be through stimulation of liver function or bile excretion as well as through an intestinal stimulation or laxative effect when the eruptions are digestive related. A vague but pragmatic term.

BOLUS: A mass of chewed food or anything resembling same.

BROMIDISM: An old-fashioned semiaddiction to bromide depressants, characterized by lethargy, loss of appetite, and similar alcoholiclike imbalances. This is a result of long-term use and is similar in pathology to chronic ingestion of Valerian. Bromides are still a common over-the-counter sedative and, although lacking the reverse glamour of heroin or barbiturate addiction, bromidism is probably just as common as ever.

BRONCHIAL DILATION: Relaxing and opening of the upper parts of the lungs to improve inspiration and relax constricting spasms.

BRONCHITIS: An infection, usually bacterial or viral, resulting in inflammation of the mucous membranes or the bronchi. Bronchitis may also be caused by chemical or allergenic agents, at least initially.

CALCULI: Kidney deposits usually of mineral salts, formed in abnormal states of the parathyroid or uric acid metabolism. Calculi, or "stones," may also be formed in the gall bladder, pancreas, and salivary glands.

CALYX: The green, clasping base of a flower.

CAPILLARY: The smallest blood or lymph vessels.

CARDIAC: Pertaining to the heart.

CARDIAC DROPSY: A generalised edema resulting from cardiac insufficiency.

CARDIAC GLYCOSIDE: Sugar-containing plant substances that, in proper doses, act as stimulants to the heart. (Example: digitalin, strophanthin.)

CARDIAC TONIC: A substance which strengthens or stimulates heart metabolism without any overt stimulation or depression, at least in moderate doses. (Example: hawthorne berries, magnesium.)

CATARRH: An inflammatory condition of any mucous membrane, usually accompanied by hypersecretion of mucous.

CATHARTIC: An energetic laxative, often causing accompanying cramps, and usually needing an antispasmodic combined with it.

CATKINS: A drooping spike formed in the spring by some plants, and most typical of the Willows.

CENTRAL NERVOUS SYSTEM: A collective term for the brain, spinal cord, their nerves, and end-organs.

CERVICAL INCOMPETENCE: A weakening of muscle tone in the cervix of the uterus making it difficult to carry full-term in pregnancy. It can be a result of frequent abortions.

CERVICITIS: An inflammation, often infectious, of the cervix of the uterus.

CERVIX: The neck and opening to the uterus.

CHOLECYSTITIS: An inflammation, usually caused by gallstones, of the gall bladder.

CHRONIC: A disease or imbalance of long, slow duration, showing little change. The opposite of acute.

CLUSTER HEADACHE: Migrainelike headaches that may occur several times a day for a week or two, usually with severe pain behind one eye. The cause is unknown, but is triggered by stress, trauma, or overwork.

COLIC: Spasms of the smooth muscles in any tube or duct. (Example: intestinal colic.)

COLITIS: An inflammation of the colon or large intestine, with or without infection.

COLONIC SPASMS: Also called irritable colon, they are characterized by alternating diarrhea and constipation, nausea, heartburn, and the like, although the spasms may or may not cause pain.

COLOSTRUM: The fluid produced by the breasts immediately following birth and for several days afterwards before milk comes in. It contains antibodies and white blood cells from the mother, as well as nutrients.

CONSTITUTION: The basic physical and emotional character of a person, including native strengths and weaknesses.

COROLLA: The petals or floral tube of a flower.

COUNTERIRRITATION: The process of applying an irritating or vasodilating substance externally to the skin in order to speed healing through local increased circulation, the radiation of heat inward to inflamed tissues from the skin, or the ill-understood reflex stimulation to seemingly unrelated internal organs. The latter, formerly used extensively by physicians but rare in recent decades due to a lack of fundamental theory, bears suspicious similarities to acupuncture and reflexology. (Example: mustard plasters.)

CYSTITIS: An inflammation of the urinary bladder, usually arising from a urethra or prostate infection below.

DECIDUOUS: A plant that drops its leaves in the fall.

DECOCTION: A tea that is boiled slowly for fifteen or twenty minutes, usually when made of roots, barks, or large seeds. Opposite of infusion.

DEMULCENT: A substance that soothes the mucous membrances on contact.

DENTATE: A leaf margin that is regularly toothed like a saw.

DIABETES INSIPIDUS: A disease characterized by constant thirst and urination caused by poor secretion of vasopressin, the antidiuretic hormone from the posterior pituitary.

DIABETES MELLITUS: A disease characterized by high blood sugar levels and sugar in the urine, caused eventually by poor secretion or utilization of insulin, but usually brought on by many years of excess sugar intake. The latter fact is still grimly resisted by many physicians.

DIAPHORETIC: A substance which increases perspiration.

DIARRHEA: A watery evacuation of the bowels, without blood.

DISTAL: Away from the center.

DIURETIC: A substance that increases the flow of urine, either by increasing permeability of the kidney cells or increasing blood flow.

DIVERTICULA: Little congenital pouches found in many organs, particularly the colon, that are benign but prone to inflammation.

DOCTRINE OF SIGNATURES: An archaic theory holding that a plant will signify its use by a "signature." By this doctrine a plant with a kidney-shaped leaf is useful in treating kidney disorders. This form of sympathetic magic is still common in many societies.

DROPSY: An older name for systemic water retention or edema.

DYSENTERY: Severe diarrhea, usually containing blood.

DYSPEPSIA: Poor digestion, usually with heartburn.

DYSPLASIA: Any abnormal tissue development.

DYSURIA: Painful urination, usually a sign of urethra, bladder, or prostate inflammation.

ECLECTICS: A former school of medicine, mostly extinct by the First World War, that used many methods of treatment in disease, empirically. Many old country doctors were trained and licensed Eclectic Physicians.

EMETIC: A substance that promotes vomiting.

EMMENAGOGUE: A substance that stimulates menstrual flow.

EMOLLIENT: A skin dressing or soothing ointment.

EMODIN: A group of related glycosides which, upon digestion in the small intestine, cause a laxative or cathartic effect. The usual plant sources are Cascara Sagrada, Buckthorn, Rhubarb, and Aloes.

ENDOCRINE: A secretion that flows directly into the bloodstream. The various unrelated endocrine glands form a sort of biochemical nervous system that is mutually interdependent.

ENDOMETRIUM: The inner mucous membrane of the uterus.

ENTIRE: A leaf with a straight, untoothed margin.

ENZYME: An organic catalyst produced by living tissue that speeds up the breakdown of other substances.

ERGOT: A poisonous fungus, *Claviceps purpurea,* that is the source of a number of clinically used substances, such as ergotamine and ergotrate.

ESTRADIOL: An estrogenic hormone secreted by the ovaries and adrenal cortex.

ESTRONE: A physiologically active estrogen byproduct.

EXOCRINE: A secretion that is external, either to mucous membranes or the skin. The opposite of endocrine.

EXPECTORANT: A substance that stimulates the outflow of mucus from the lungs and bronchials.

FEBRILE: Feverish.

FERAL: Wild, native.

FIXED OILS: Oils that leave a residue and do not evaporate. (Example: olive oil.)

FOMENTATION: A hot, wet poultice used on painful, inflamed areas. The usual form is a towel dipped in tea and applied, being changed when it cools.

FUNGICIDE: A substance that kills or inhibits fungus infections.

GALENIC: Referring to the ancient physician, Galen. Loosely applied to unrefined plant medications.

GASTRITIS: Inflammation of the stomach.

GASTROENTERITIS: Inflammation of the stomach and intestines. "Stomach Flu."

GLABROUS: A plant having no hairs.

GLAUCOUS: Hairless and possessing a bloom, like Concord grapes.

GLYCOSIDE: A plant substance that, upon hydrolysis, is broken into a sugar and one or more other substances.

GLYCOSURIA: The presence of sugar (glucose) in the urine.

GOUT: A joint inflammation, usually of the knee or foot, resulting from deposits of urea salts.

HEMATURIA: The presence of blood in the urine.

HEMOSTATIC: A substance which stops bleeding, internally or externally.

HEPATIC DUCT: The bile duct from the liver that bypasses the gall bladder and, with it, empties into the common bile duct, thence into the duodenum.

HEPATITIS: An inflammation of the liver. It may have many causes, only one of which is the hepatitis virus.

HIATUS HERNIA: A protrusion of the stomach through the diaphragm wall, common in middle-aged women.

HOMEOPATHY: A biochemical approach to medicine which works from the premise that a substance taken in large doses by a healthy individual will be useful, in minute doses, in curing the same symptoms that substance produced, in a sick individual. Although homeopathic medicines are by no means harmless, they are completely devoid of drug toxicity, and the practice is widespread throughout the world. In the U.S., however, only perhaps a hundred physicians are predominantly homeopathic. Traditionally, homeopathy acknowedges no diseases, only symptoms.

HYPERURICEMIA: An abnormal amount of uric acid in the blood. This often can lead to gout and kidney stones.

IDIOPATHIC: A fancy garbage-bag term used in medicine to denote a condition or disease of unknown origin.

ILEO-CECAL VALVE: The valve or sphincter that separates the ileum part of the small intestine from the ascending colon.

ILEUM: The lower two-thirds of the small intestine, ending in the ileo-cecal valve.

INFUSION: A method of brewing tea in which boiling water is poured over a plant, usually reserved for leaves, flowers, and small seeds. The opposite of decoction.

KERATOLYTIC: A substance which loosens or dissolves horny layers of the skin. (Example: Corn plaster, salicylic acid.)

KERATOSIS PILARIS: An inflammatory condition of the skin surrounding hair follicles.

LANCEOLATE: A leaf that is lance shaped.

LOCHIA: The cleansing drainage from the uterus following childbirth.

LYMPHATIC: Pertaining to the lymph system or lymph tissue, the "back alley" of the body. Lymph is the alkaline, clear intercellular fluid that drains from soft tissue, is filtered by the lymph nodes, and eventually is cycled into the veins of the upper chest. Lymph nodes in the small intestine absorb most of the fats from food, which often makes postintestinal lymph milky. Lymph nodes and lymph tissue in the spleen, thymus, and tonsils also form the lymphocytes, hyperactive white blood corpuscles that scavenge the soft tissues and manufacture antibodies.

LYRATE: A leaf that is lyre shaped.

MANNITE: An indigestible starch used, as mannitol, to facilitate other diuretics in medical practice. Found, often with inulin, in Dandelion roots and other roots of the Compositeae family of plants.

MASTITIS: Inflammation or infection of the breast.

MERIDIANS: Nonphysical energy pathways used in oriental and recent western therapies to diagnose and stimulate healing of internal organ or systemic imbalances. Meridian diagnosis and therapy is a large part of present as well as historical oriental medicine, and plays a major role in newer chiropractice as well as reflexology, "acupressure," and such.

METABOLITE: Any by-product of metabolism.

MONILIA: A "yeast," common to the vagina and mouth.

MONONUCLEOSIS: In common use, a virus infection of the lymph tissue, characterized by enlarged nodes, spleen, and, sometimes, liver.

MUCILAGE: A number of plant substances characterized by thick, slimy viscosity. Often used as emollients or demulcents.

MULTIPLE SCLEROSIS: A chronic disease characterized by a breakdown in the protective cells of the nervous system. Contrary to popular opinion, it can totally remiss, or disappear for years, and cortisone therapy can never cure the disease, only lessen symptoms and prolong the course.

NARCOTIC: A substance that depresses central nervous system function, bringing sleep and lessening pain. By definition, narcotics can be toxic in excess.

NATUROPATHY: A medical system that uses many and varied methods, including herbs, to bring about the body's health through stimulating its innate defense mechanisms, never supplanting them with drugs. The basis of naturopathy is facilitating a "healing crisis" through hydrotherapy, massage, heat, herbs, and whatever means are handy. The practice almost disappeared in the 1950s, with many unscrupulous individuals practicing or selling mail-order degrees, but has made a respectable comeback recently, primarily because of several four-year residency schools and an increased pressure for licensing and state-recognised criteria.

NEPHRITIS: An inflammation of the kidneys.

NERVINE: A substance that quells nervousness and irritability, either through depression or stimulation of the central nervous system.

NEURALGIA: Pain, sometimes severe, manifest along the length of a nerve, often having no detectable effects other than the pain.

OPPOSITE: Having the leaves arranged in pairs along opposite sides of the stem.

ORCHITIS: Inflammation of one or both testicles.

OVAL-LANCEOLATE: A leaf that is longer than wide but somewhat rounded in the center.

OXYTOCIC: A substance that stimulates uterine contractions.

PALLIATIVE: Relieving symptoms without affecting the cause.

PALMATE: A hand-shaped leaf.

PARASYMPATHETIC: A division of the autonomic (automatic) nervous system that controls normal digestive, reproductive, and cardiopulmonary function, as well as stimulating secretions other than sweat. Sometimes called the "yin" influence of the nervous system.

PARASYMPATHOMIMETIC: A substance that mimics parasympathetic function.

PARTURITION: Childbirth.

PEDICEL: A stem holding a single flower, either solitary or clustered.

PEDUNCLE: A stem holding a flower cluster.

PERISTALSIS: The rhythmical wavelike contractions of smooth muscles, usually in reference to the intestinal tract.

PHENOLS: A group of aromatic benzene derivatives having bacteriostatic effects in small amounts, corrosive effects in large amounts.

PHOSPHATES: Salts of phosphoric acid, critical in maintaining a proper acid-alkaline balance in the blood, where they help neutralize waste products.

PHYSIOLOGICAL DOSE: An amount of a substance sufficient to cause a physical effect, as opposed to the minute quantities in attenuation of the substance used homeopathically.

PHYTOSTEROLS: A sterol, or fatty alcohol, found in many forms in plants.

PINNATE: A compound leaf having the leaflets arranged on either side of the stem or petiole. (Example: Sweet Pea.)

PLEURISY: Inflammation of the membrane that enfolds the lungs.

POST PARTUM: After childbirth.

POULTICE: A hot, moist mass, consisting of a base (slippery elm, comfrey root, clay, flax seed, kudzu, bran, etc.) and one or more active substances (mustard seed, ginger, anemone, etc.) and placed on any part of the body, held (usually) between two pieces of muslin, and changed when cool. This aids pain, congestive inflammation, and tissue damage, as well as speeding absorption into the poultice of waste products, protein metabolites, and free amino acids.

PREECLAMPSIA: A condition of pregnancy resulting in water retention in the legs, high blood pressure, headache, and poor kidney function. Commonly called toxemia, it can progress into eclampsia and should be monitered carefully.

PROLAPSED UTERUS: A lowered displacement of the uterus, with the cervix protruding downward into the vagina.

PROSTATITIS: An inflammation of the prostate gland, a doughnut-shaped gland secreting semen fluids that surround the juncture of the urethra and the bladder.

PROTEOLYTIC ENZYME: An enzyme that speeds up the breaking down of proteins.

PSORIASIS: A patchy dermatitis, usually of chronic nature and often inherited, especially in those with thin skin.

PULMONARY EDEMA: A collecting of fluids in the lungs, usually due to inflammation or poor circulation and drainage.

PURINE: A protein metabolite, often derived from cellular digestion, and breaking down into uric acid. Some alkaloids, such as caffeine, contain purines.

PYOGENIC MEMBRANE: A membrane formed, or remaining, over an infection that forms pus.

RACEME: An elongated, terminal flowering stem. (Example: Lavender.)

REFLEXED: Bent backwards, away from the direction of growth.

RENAL: Of the kidneys.

RESIN: A gummy, oily secretion or residue in a plant. (Example: pitch.)

RESTORATIVE: A substance that stimulates a return, after disease, to normal function and metabolism.

RHIZOME: A creeping horizontal root that gives rise to several stems.

RUBIFACIENT: A substance that dilates the skin, bringing a greater blood supply to the area. If blistering occurs it is termed vesicant.

SACRAL NERVES: Five pairs of nerves, both motor and sensory, that emerge from the base of the spinal chord (sacrum and coccyx).

SALICYLATES: Broadly speaking, salicylic acid and its salts, as well as aspirin. All are useful in reducing pain and inflammation, and all act as counterirritants. Oil of Wintergreen (methyl salicylate) should only be used externally, however.

SAPOGENINS: Soapy-oily plant substances used as precursors to the manufacturing of steroids, some having physiological actions.

SAPONINS: Soapy glycosides found in the roots of some plants, usually having an irritating effect on the intestinal mucosa.

SEBACEOUS GLANDS: The oil-secreting glands of the skin, most surrounding hair follicles.

SEDATIVE: Sleep inducing.

SEPAL: A leaf or segment of the calyx.

SEPTICEMIA: The presence of disease-causing bacteria in the bloodstream, potentially fatal.

SEROUS: Membranes inside the body that secrete serum as a lubricant. (Example: The pleura of the lungs.)

SERRATED: Saw-toothed margins of leaves that point forward, as opposed to dentate, which point outward.

SITZ BATH: A cleansing or therapeutic bath in a small tub, holding enough water to sit in with the hips covered and the legs and torso above water.

SKELETAL MUSCLES: Also called striped muscles or voluntary muscles, they are subject to conscious control.

SMOOTH MUSCLES: Also called involuntary muscles, they are under the control of the autonomic nervous system and are (supposedly) not under conscious control.

SPLEEN: The large organ lying to the left, below, and behind the stomach, which is partially responsible for white blood cell formation (red, in childhood), the storage and concentration of red blood cells and the ejection of them by contraction under stress, and the filtering and removing of flotsum and old red blood cells.

STEROIDS: Specifically, the hormones of the adrenal cortex and the gonads; broadly, any number of fatty compounds such as bile acids, Vitamin D, and phytosterols.

STIPULE: Little appendage formed at the juncture of a leaf and the main plant stem.

SUBALPINE: Directly below timberline; high mountain forest.

SUPPURATING: Infected and discharging pus, or more broadly, sloughing off of tissue.

SYDENHAM'S CHOREA: Irregular palsy of the face and limbs, often a self-limiting syndrome of children.

SYMPATHETIC: A division of the autonomic or involuntary nervous system that lacks selective function and works only *in toto,* usually in conjunction with the adrenal medulla. The nerve endings secrete a substance similar to adrenalin, and as the adrenal medulla secretes that hormone, to varying degrees, all of the muscles that react to the sympathetic nerves also react to adrenalin. Typified by "yang" energies, a chronic excess of sympathetic function (called stress) is the major contributing factor to most of the diseases of older Americans. Since one of the first subjective symptoms of subclinical malnutrition is irritability, hypersympathetic functions act as an intermediate between chronic poor diet and disease.

SYMPATHOMIMETIC: A substance that mimics adrenalin (epinephrine). (Example: Ephedrine, amphetamines, caffeine.)

SYSTEMIC: Reacting on the body as a whole, as opposed to a single tissue and, by inference, carried in the bloodstream.

SYSTOLIC: The measurement of blood pressure at the point of heart contraction, as opposed to diastolic, which is the measurement at rest.

TACHYCARDIA: Abnormally fast heart beat.

TANNINS: Protective substances found in the outer and inner tissues of plants that form undigestible substances to animals, breaking down through age to phlebotannins and finally humin, all undigestible and protecting the plants from infection and such. All act on tissue as astringents, but differ in chemistry and accompanying substances. Tannin-containing plants can vary a great deal in their physiological effects and should not be lumped together (as they often are).

TENESMUS: Painful spasmodic contractions of intestinal muscles, usually of the large intestine, rectum. and anus.

TINCTURE: A water and alcohol concentration of a plant, used either for convenience, i.e., external application, or because some of the active constituents are not very soluble in tea. If the fresh plant has been juiced or puréed, ten percent grain alcohol or twenty-five percent vodka may be added to preserve. Otherwise, in a dried plant, twice the volume of the ground herb in vodka is added to it, steeped for at least ten days, and the whole mass expressed through a press or wrung out by hand through a cloth. Variations from plant to plant are noted in the text. Tinctures should be stored in amber bottles if possible and kept out of direct light. Vinegar may be used as a solvent (menstruum) but is sometimes inferior in extraction of oils.

TONIC: A substance taken to strengthen, usually in the absence of disease. A preventative herb.

TOXEMIA: Autotoxicity, either through septicemia and the systemic distribution of bacterial exotoxins or through the breakdown of some excretory functions and a recycling of waste products in the blood.

TOXINS: Poisonous substances of external or internal nature. The disease reactions to many microorganisms is often due to their toxic waste products and not the presence, per se, of the parasite. Fever, lethargy, and inflammations are some reactions, defensive in nature, that the body can manifest in the presence of excess toxin levels.

TRIGEMINAL NEURALGIA: Tic douloureux. Nerve pain, sometimes with loss of motor control, of the trigeminal nerve controlling the side of the the face.

TRIGONE: The triangular muscle at the base of the bladder, extending from the two ureter openings to the urethra opening.

TRIMESTER: The three three-month divisions of a nine-month pregnancy.

TUBER: The thick, underground stems or roots of many plants, often with buds present.

UMBEL: A flower or seed formation, where the stems radiate to each flower like the supports in an upended umbrella. (Example: Celery.)

URETHRA: The canal between the bladder and the outside of the body.

URETHRITIS: An inflammation of the urethra.

URIC ACID: The final end product of protein or nitrogenous breakdown and metabolism in the body. Since it cannot break down further under normal circumstances, it is excreted primarily in the urine and sweat.

UVULA: The small structure in the back of the throat that hangs down from the palate.

VAGINISMUS: A spasm of the vaginal muscles, usually from trauma or an emotional aversion to sexual intercourse. Very painful and not controllable voluntarily.

VAGINITIS: An inflammation of the vaginal canal.

VAGUS NERVE: The pneumogastric or tenth cranial nerve, and a major portion of parasympathetic enervation, as well as the largest cranial nerve.

VASOCONSTRICTOR: A substance that causes a narrowing or constriction of blood vessels.

VASODILATOR: A substance that causes a relaxing and dilation of blood vessels.

VERMICIDE: A substance that kills or expels intestinal worms.

VILLI: The little hairs or filaments found on many membranes, often to increase surface area, as in the small intestine.

VOLATILE OILS: Those oils which evaporate and leave no residue.

VULNERARY: A first aid for wounds and skin abrasions.

XEROPHYTE: A plant that is drought resistant or is found in the desert.

THERAPEUTIC and USE INDEX

This is an index only.
Please refer to the main text for specific information before using any herb.

ABORTIVE
Inmortal
Mistletoe
Pennyroyal
Peony

ALCOHOLISM
Dogbane
Hops
Oshá
Skullcap

ALTERATIVE
Barberry
Blue Flag
Burdock
Figwort
Inmortal
Oregon Grape
Oshá
Red Clover
Toadflax
Yellow Dock

ANALGESIC
Birch
California Bay
California Poppy
Cocklebur
Cow Parsnip
Hops
Jimson Weed (external)
Lobelia
Poplar
Prickly Poppy
Skullcap
Tobacco (external)
Valerian
Willow

ANTI-INFLAMMATORY (Systemic)
Agave
Barberry
Birch
Gentian
Hop Tree
Licorice
Oregon Grape
Poplar
Sweet Clover
Willow

ANTISEPTIC
Alum Root
Barberry
Betony
Bistort
Blue Flag
Cañaigre
Cocklebur
Cranesbill
Hops
Oregon Grape
Oshá
Tobacco
Willow

ANTISPASMODIC
Angelica
Betony
Catnip
Cocklebur
Corydalis
Evening Primrose
Marsh Marigold
Mistletoe
St. John's Wort
Tobacco (external)
Valerian
Vervain

With Laxatives
Angelica
Bayberry
California Bay
Cow Parsnip
Oshá

APHRODISIAC
Broomrape (?)
Dodder (?)

APPETITE DEPRESSANT
Maravilla

APPETITE STIMULANT
Gentian
Hops
Poplar

ARTHRITIS
External

Apache Plume
Arnica
Escoba de la Víbora
Jimson Weed
Lobelia
Maravilla
Poplar
Storksbill
Tobacco
See COUNTERIRRITANT,
   POULTICE

Internal
Agave
Alfalfa
Birch
Cocklebur
Coffee Berry
Cota
Dogbane
Escoba de la Víbora
Hop Tree
Licorice
Poplar
Storksbill
Willow
Yucca
See ANALGESIC,
   ANTI-INFLAMMATORY,
   MUSCLE/JOINT

ASTRINGENT
Agrimony
Alum Root
Amaranth
Avens
Betony
Bistort
Broomrape
Cañaigre
Cat's Paw
Contrayerba
Cranesbill
Manzanita
Mormon Tea
Nettles
Oak
Potentilla
Self Heal
Storksbill
Uva Ursi

BEER MAKING
Hop Tree

183

Hops
Horehound

BLOOD SUGAR

Blueberry
Maravilla

BROOMS

Grindelia

CANCER

Cleavers
Yellow Dock

CAPILLARY FRAGILITY

Oak

CARDIAC STIMULANT

Burning Bush
Coneflower
Dogbane
False Solomon's Seal (?)
Inmortal

CARDIAC TONIC

Grindelia (relaxant)
Inmortal
Motherwort

CELIAC DISEASE

Alfalfa

CHEWING GUM

Grindelia
Pine
Yerba Santa

CHOREA (Palsy)

Corydalis
Skullcap

COLDS/FLU

Bayberry
Elder
Inmortal
Mormon Tea
Oshá
Pennyroyal
Red Root
Sage
Vervain
Willow
Yerba Santa
See EXPECTORANT,
  RESPIRATORY SYSTEM,
  SINUSES, THROAT
  INFLAMMATION

COLIC

Amaranth
Catnip

Hops
Pennyroyal
Poleo
Spearmint
Vervain

CONVALESCENT AID

Alfalfa
Juniper (aroma)
Mallow
Red Clover
Spearmint
Strawberry
Sweet Clover (aroma)
See RESTORATIVE

COUGH

Demulcent

Apache Plume
False Solomon's Seal
Fremontia
Hound's Tongue
Maidenhair
Mallow
Yerba de la Negrita

Suppressant

Bayberry
Horehound
Lobelia
Mullein
Red Clover
See EXPECTORANT,
  LARYNGITIS, RESPIRATORY
  SYSTEM, THROAT
  INFLAMMATION

COUNTERIRRITANT

Arnica
Baneberry
Birch
Clematis
Cow Parsnip
Dogbane
Maravilla
Marsh Marigold
Pipsissewa
Poplar
Pyrola
Tobacco
Willow
See POULTICE

DEMULCENT-EMOLLIENT

False Solomon's Seal
Fremontia
Hound's Tongue
Mallow
Plantain
Rattlesnake Plantain
Yerba de la Negrita

DIAPHORETIC

Angelica
Betony
Blue Curls
Blue Flag
Dogbane
Elder
Horehound
Inmortal
Juniper
Oregano de la Sierra
Oshá
Pennyroyal
Pleurisy Root
Poleo
Spearmint
Vervain
Wormwood
Yarrow

Antidiaphoretic

Sage
See FEVER

DIET AID

Change of

Blue Flag

Minerals

Nettles
Red Clover

Vitamins

Alfalfa
Nettles
Oak

DIURETIC

Asparagus
Birch
Blue Flag
Burdock
Burning Bush
Cachana
Chicory
Cleavers
Cocklebur
Coneflower
Dandelion
Dogbane
Elder
Evening Primrose
Horsetail
Mallow
Milkweed
Mormon Tea
Mullein
Oregano de la Sierra
Storksbill
Strawberry
Vervain
Willow

Disinfecting

Blueberry
Burdock (seed)
Cota
Grindelia
Juniper
Manzanita
Pine
Pipsissewa
Poplar
Pyrola
Uva Ursi
Yerba Santa
See URINARY TRACT

DOUCHE

Alum Root
Amaranth
Cat's Paw
Cranesbill
Manzanita
Nettles
Plantain
Self Heal
Storksbill
Strawberry
Uva Ursi

DRUG ADJUNCT

Alfalfa
Clematis
Licorice

EARACHE

Mullein

ENDOCRINE SYSTEM

Steroidal

Agave
Angelica
Cow Parsnip
Licorice
Oshá
Yucca

Thyroid

Bugleweed (depressant)
Oregon Grape (stimulant)
See REPRODUCTIVE
   SYSTEM—FEMALE, MALE

ENEMA

Alum Root
Catnip
Cat's Paw
Cranesbill
Nettles
Oak
Strawberry

EXPECTORANT

Bayberry

Burning Bush
False Solomon's Seal
Grindelia
Horehound
Inmortal
Lobelia
Mallow
Marsh Marigold
Milkweed
Oshá
Pine
Pleurisy Root
Red Clover
St. John's Wort
Yerba Santa
See RESPIRATORY SYSTEM

EYES

Agrimony
Contrayerba
Prickly Poppy (?)
Rattlesnake Plantain
Red Root
Self Heal

FAINTING/ DIZZINESS

California Bay
Pennyroyal

FEET

Potentilla
Tobacco
Yerba de la Negrita

FEVER

Sedative

Angelica
Coral Root
Tobacco (external)
Vervain

Stimulant

Angelica
Blue Curls
Cota
Elder
Oshá
Pennyroyal
Poleo
Wormwood
Yarrow
See DIAPHORETIC

Suppressant

Barberry
Birch
Gentian
Hop Tree
Oregon Grape
Poplar
Potentilla
Raspberry

Self Heal
Willow

FISHING

Amole Lily

FLORAL DÉCORATION

Cachana (flowers)
Maidenhair
Yarrow

FOOD

Amaranth
Angelica
Asparagus
Barberry
Elderberry
Evening Primrose
Hops
Licorice
Manzanita
Marsh Marigold
Nettles
Plantain
Prickly Poppy
Raspberry
Strawberry
See SPICE, TEA

FUNGICIDE

Cebadilla
Figwort
Prickly Poppy
Tobacco

HAIR

Dandruff

Amole Lily
Yerba de la Negrita
Yucca

Growth Stimulant

Apache Plume
Birch
Dogbane
Nettles
Red Root
Willow

Rinse

Maidenhair
Yarrow
Yerba de la Negrita
Yucca
See SOAP/SHAMPOO

HEADACHE

Birch
Cachana
California Bay
Clematis
False Solomon's Seal

Pennyroyal
Poplar
Self Heal
Tobacco (poultice)
Willow
See ANALGESIC

HEMORRHOIDS

Amaranth
Hound's Tongue
Jimson Weed (external)
Red Root
Tobacco (external)
Yarrow
Yellow Dock
Yerba de la Negrita

HEMOSTATIC

Alum Root
Bistort
Bugleweed
Cañaigre
Cocklebur
Contrayerba
Cranesbill
Horsetail
Mistletoe
Nettles
Oak
Self Heal
Yarrow

HYPERTENSION

Oshá
Skullcap
Valerian
See CARDIAC TONIC, DIURETIC,
  NERVOUS SYSTEM,
  SEDATIVE/TRANQUILIZER

HYPERURICEMIA

Asparagus
See DIURETIC, MUSCLE/JOINT,
  URINARY TRACT

INFECTION— LOCAL

See ANTISEPTIC, SKIN, various
  headings

INFECTION— SYSTEMIC

Angelica
Blue Flag
Oshá
See FEVER

INSECT REPELLENT

Mountain Mahogany
Oshá
Pennyroyal
Poleo

INSECTICIDE

Tobacco

INTESTINAL TRACT

Colitis

Alfalfa
Contrayerba
Cow Parsnip
Cranesbill
Plantain
Sweet Clover

Cramps, Tenesmus

Angelica
Bayberry
California Bay
Cow Parsnip
Oshá
Sweet Clover
Valerian
See ANTISPASMODIC

Diarrhea/Dysentery

Alum Root
Amaranth
Avens
Bayberry
Bistort
California Bay
Cocklebur
Contrayerba
Nettles
Plantain
Poplar
Potentilla
Raspberry
Rose
Sage
Self Heal
Strawberry
Wormwood
See ENEMA

Inflammation, Small Intestine

Alum Root
Amaranth
Cat's Paw
Contrayerba
Cranesbill
Gentian
Hound's Tongue
Plantain
Sage
Sweet Clover
Wormwood
Yerba de la Negrita

Tonic

Barberry
Gentian
Hop Tree

Horehound
Oregon Grape
Oshá
Poplar
Wormwood

Ulcers

Alfalfa
Bistort
Cranesbill
Hound's Tongue
Plantain
Red Root
See LAXATIVE/CATHARTIC,
  LIVER (BILE AND
  GALL BLADDER STIMULANT),
  PANCREAS, STOMACH

LARYNGITIS

False Solomon's Seal
Fremontia
Hound's Tongue
Maidenhair
Mallow

LAXATIVE/ CATHARTIC

Agave
Asparagus
Barberry
Blue Flag
Broomrape
Burning Bush
Cebadilla
Chicory
Coffee Berry
Dandelion
Dodder
Elder
Evening Primrose
Inmortal
Licorice
Maravilla
Mountain Mahogany
Oregon Grape
Prickly Poppy (seeds)
Yarrow
Yellow Dock
Yucca
See ANTISPASMODIC (to
  prevent gripping)

Lubricating

Licorice
Plantain (seeds)

LIVER

Bile and Gall Bladder Stimulant

Barberry
Blue Flag
Burning Bush

Cat's Paw　　　　　＼
Coffee Berry
Oregon Grape
Toadflax
Yellow Dock

Hepatitis

Cleavers
Dandelion
Red Clover

Jaundice

Agave
Toadflax
Yellow Dock

Post-Hepatitis

Barberry
Cat's Paw
Oregon Grape
Toadflax
Yellow Dock

Tonic/Stimulant

Barberry
Blue Flag
Burning Bush
Cachana
Cat's Paw
Chicory
Cleavers
Coffee Berry
Dandelion
Dodder
Hop Tree
Oregon Grape
Toadflax
Yellow Dock
See ALTERATIVE, SKIN
(Irruptions)

LYMPHATIC STIMULANT

Bayberry
Blue Flag
Dodder
Inmortal
Oregon Grape
Pleurisy Root
Red Clover
Red Root
See SPLEEN

MAGIC-TALISMAN-RITUAL

Cachana
Jimson Weed
Juniper
Maravilla
Oshá
Tobacco
Yarrow

MERIDIAN DIAGNOSIS

Red Root
Vervain

MOUTH-GUM INFLAMMATION

Barberry
Bistort
Cañaigre
Contrayerba
Cranesbill
-Oak
Oregon Grape
Potentilla
Self Heal
Strawberry

Toothache, Topical

Cow Parsnip
Cranesbill
Oak
Oshá
Tobacco

MUSCLE/JOINT

Arnica
Asparagus (gout)
Birch
Blueberry (gout)
Burdock (seed)
Contrayerba
Cow Parsnip
Hop Tree
Jimson Weed (external)
Lobelia (external)
Poplar
Tobacco (external)
Willow
See ANALGESIC,
ANTI-INFLAMMATORY,
ARTHRITIS,
COUNTERIRRITANT, POULTICE

MUSCLE RELAXANT

Betony
Evening Primrose
Lobelia
Mistletoe
Motherwort
Skullcap
See ANTISPASMODIC,
SEDATIVE/TRANQUILIZER

NERVOUS SYSTEM

Epilepsy

Skullcap

Herpes Zoster or Shingles

Motherwort

Nervine/Tonic

Bugleweed

Corydalis
Peony
Skullcap
Valerian

Neuralgia

California Bay
Cow Parsnip
Skullcap
Valerian

Paralysis

Cow Parsnip

Parasympathomimetic

Blue Flag
Dogbane
Elder
Inmortal
Lobelia
Milkweed
Peony
Pleurisy Root
See ANTISPASMODIC, CHOREA,
MUSCLE RELAXANT,
SEDATIVE/TRANQUILIZER,
STIMULANT

NOSEBLEED

Bugleweed
Cachana
Red Root

PANCREAS

Barberry
Blue Flag
Hop Tree
Marsh Marigold
Oregon Grape
Yellow Dock

PARASITES

Body

Cebadilla
Jimson Weed
Larkspur
Tobacco

Intestinal

Hop Tree
Wormwood

PERSONAL HYGIENE

Mullein Leaves

PILLOWS

Sweet Clover
Wormwood

POLISHING

Horsetail

POULTICE

Apache Plume

Bistort
Broomrape
Cow Parsnip
Fremontia
Hound's Tongue
Jimson Weed (external)
Lobelia
Mallow
Maravilla
Marsh Marigold
Plantain
Poplar
Potentilla
Prickly Poppy
Self Heal
Tobacco
Willow
Yerba de la Negrita
See ARTHRITIS,
  COUNTERIRRITANT,
  DEMULCENT-EMOLLIENT

PREGNANCY/
POSTPARTUM
Labor

Blue Curls
Inmortal
Mallow
Mistletoe
Pennyroyal
Poleo
Spearmint

Lactation

Inmortal (stimulant)
Sage (depressant)

Mastitis

Red Root
Sweet Clover
See REPRODUCTIVE
  SYSTEM—FEMALE

Postpartum

Bugleweed
Coral Root
Cranesbill
Inmortal
Manzanita
Motherwort
Oshá
Self Heal
Uva Ursi

Pre-eclampsia

Burdock (seed)

Tonic

Alfalfa
Raspberry
Strawberry

RENNET (Vegetable)

Nettles
Sweet Clover

REPRODUCTIVE
SYSTEM—FEMALE
Antimenstrual

Avens
Broomrape
Bugleweed
Contrayerba
Cranesbill
Escoba de la Víbora
Horsetail
Manzanita
Nettles
Peony
Raspberry
Red Root
Sage
Self Heal
Storksbill
Strawberry
Uva Ursi
Yarrow

Cramps

Angelica
Coneflower
Cow Parsnip
Evening Primrose
Inmortal
Licorice
Motherwort
Pennyroyal
Peony
Poleo
Raspberry
Storksbill
Tobacco (poultice)
Uva Ursi
Wormwood

Menopause

Broomrape
Licorice

Prolapsed Uterus

Burdock
See ANTISPASMODIC, DOUCHE,
  PREGNANCY/POSTPARTUM

Promenstrual

Angelica
Blue Curls
Cow Parsnip
Inmortal
Maidenhair
Motherwort
Oregano de la Sierra
Pennyroyal
Peony
Poleo
Wormwood

Vaginal Discharge

Avens
Cranesbill

Inmortal
Nettles
Raspberry

Vaginismus

Motherwort

Vaginitis/Cervicitis

Alum
Amaranth
Cranesbill
Manzanita (sitz bath)
Nettles
Plantain
Storksbill
Uva Ursi (sitz bath)

REPRODUCTIVE
SYSTEM—MALE
Orchitis

Peony

Prostitis

Barberry
Bugleweed
Mountain Mahogany
Oregon Grape
Peony
Raspberry
Yucca

RESPIRATORY
SYSTEM
Asthma

Cow Parsnip
Grindelia
Horehound
Inmortal
Jimson Weed (smoked)
Licorice
Lobelia
Mormon Tea
Mullein
Valerian
Yerba Santa

Bronchitis/"Chest Colds"

Grindelia
Horehound
Jimson Weed (smoked)
Licorice
Maidenhair
Mormon Tea
Mullein
Nettles
Plantain
Pleurisy Root
Yerba Santa
See COLDS/FLU, COUGH,
  EXPECTORANT, LARYNGITIS,
  SINUSES, THROAT
  INFLAMMATION, TONSILLITIS

Pleurisy

Inmortal

Licorice
Milkweed
Pleurisy Root
Yerba Santa

RESTORATIVE
Alfalfa
Broomrape
Cota
Gentian
Oshá
Red Clover
Skullcap

SALIVA
Depressant
Cañaigre
Jimson Weed
Sage

Stimulant
Cebadilla
Gentian
Inmortal
Oshá
Pleurisy Root

SAUNA HERBS
Juniper
Pine
Wormwood

SEDATIVE/ TRANQUILIZER
Betony
Broomrape
Bugleweed
California Poppy
Catnip
Coral Root
Evening Primrose
Figwort
Grindelia
Hops
Horsetail
Lobelia
Peony
Prickly Poppy
Red Clover
Skullcap
St. John's Wort
Valerian
Vervain

SINUSES
Bayberry
Inmortal
Marsh Marigold
Mormon Tea
Oshá
Pleurisy Root
Red Root
Sage

Yerba Santa
See COLDS/FLU

SKIN
Abrasions/Cuts
Agave
Alum Root
Barberry
Bistort
Cañaigre
Cranesbill
Manzanita
Oak
Oregon Grape
Oshá
Penstemon
Pine
Plantain
Poplar
Potentilla
Prickly Poppy
Rattlesnake Plantain
Self Heal
St. John's Wort
Uva Ursi
Willow
See ASTRINGENTS, HEMOSTATICS

Burns
Agave
Bistort
Cañaigre
Cleavers
Cranesbill
Figwort
Fremontia
Hound's Tongue
Jimson Weed
Mallow
Oak
Penstemon
Poplar
Potentilla
Prickly Poppy
Tobacco
See ANALGESIC, ASTRINGENT, DEMULCENT-EMOLLIENT

Irruptions, Internal Causes
Burdock
Figwort
Pipsissewa
Pyrola
Yellow Dock
See ALTERATIVE, LIVER, LYMPHATIC STIMULANT

Keratolytic
Burdock
Cranesbill
Inmortal (sap)
Milkweed (sap)
Plantain (fresh)

Yellow Dock

Poison Oak
Grindelia
Potentilla
Wormwood
Yerba Santa

Rashes/Dermatitis
Agrimony
Amole Lily
Bistort
Cota
Cranesbill
Figwort
Fremontia
Mallow
Manzanita
Oak
Oshá
Penstemon
Plantain
Poplar
Potentilla
Prickly Poppy
Rattlesnake Plantain
Self Heal
St. John's Wort
Uva Ursi
Willow
Yerba de la Negrita

Staph Infection
Barberry
Blue Flag
Hops
Oregon Grape
Oshá
Willow
Yellow Dock
See INFECTION—SYSTEMIC

Ulceration
Cleavers
Cranesbill
Fremontia
Hops
Hound's Tongue
Mallow
Manzanita
Oak
Penstemon
Plantain
Uva Ursi
Willow
Yellow Dock
Yerba de la Negrita
See POULTICE

Warts
Milkweed (sap)
Prickly Poppy

SMOKING, HERBS FOR

Jimson Weed (asthma)
Lobelia (asthma)
Manzanita
Mullein
Prickly Poppy (intoxicant)
Raspberry
Spearmint
Strawberry
Sweet Clover
Tobacco
Uva Ursi
Willow (bark)
Yerba Santa

SMOKING SUBSTITUTE

Licorice
Lobelia (tea)
Oshá

SOAP/SHAMPOO

Agave
Amole Lily
Bayberry (oil for making)
Red Root (flowers)
Yucca

SPICE

Angelica (leaf, seed)
Bayberry
California Bay
Juniper
Oregano de la Sierra
Oshá (leaf, seed)
Poleo (cake lining)
Sage
Sweet Clover (vodka, wine, cheese)
Wormwood
See FOOD, RENNET
(Vegetable), TEA

SPLEEN

Dandelion
Dodder
Red Root
See LYMPHATIC STIMULANT

STIMULANT

Maravilla
Mormon Tea
Oshá
Red Root (leaf)
Yerba Santa

STOMACH

Bitter Tonic

Barberry
Cebadilla
Gentian

Grindelia
Hop Tree
Hops
Horehound
Oregon Grape
Oshá
Poplar
Sage
Vervain
Wormwood
Yarrow

Cramps

Angelica
Catnip
Hops
Poleo
Spearmint
Valerian
Yarrow

Gas, Fermentation

Agave
Angelica
Cow Parsnip
Hops
Juniper
Oshá
Pennyroyal
Poleo
Spearmint
Sweet Clover
Wormwood

Hiatus Hernia

Cow Parsnip

Hiccups

Catnip
Hops

Indigestion, Dyspepsia

Agave
Apache Plume
Avens
Bayberry
Blue Curls
Bugleweed
Catnip
Cota
Cow Parsnip
Cranesbill
Escoba de la Víbora
False Solomon's Seal
Gentian
Hop Tree
Hops
Juniper
Mallow
Oregon Grape
Oshá
Pennyroyal
Poleo
Poplar

Self Heal
Spearmint
Strawberry
Sweet Clover
Vervain
Wormwood
Yarrow

Ulcers

Alum Root
Avens
Bayberry
Bistort
Cranesbill
Fremontia
Hound's Tongue
Licorice
Mallow
Poleo
Potentilla
Red Root
Sage
Self Heal
Yerba de la Negrita

TANNING

Cañaigre
Manzanita
Mormon Tea
Uva Ursis

TEA (For the Taste)

Bayberry (leaf)
Blue Curls
Chicory
Cota
Grindelia (leaf)
Mallow
Mormon Tea
Nettles (leaf)
Pennyroyal
Pine (needles)
Poleo
Red Clover
Red Root (leaf)
Self Heal
Spearmint
Strawberry
Sweet Clover

THROAT INFLAMMATION

Alum Root
Bistort
Cachana
Cranesbill
Evening Primrose
False Solomon's Seal
Fremontia
Horehound
Hound's Tongue
Licorice
Mallow

Mullein
Oregano de la Sierra
Oshá
Potentilla
Red Root
Sage
Self Heal
Yerba de la Negrita
Yerba Santa
See COUGH,
  DEMULCENT-EMOLLIENT,
  LARYNGITIS, RESPIRATORY
  SYSTEM, TONSILLITIS

TIC DOULOUREUX
Cow Parsnip
Marsh Marigold
See ANALGESIC,
  COUNTERIRRITANT, MUSCLE
  RELAXANT, NERVOUS SYSTEM
(Neuralgia)

TONSILLITIS
Cachana
Cranesbill
Mallow
Potentilla
Red Root
Sage

URINARY TRACT
Cystitis/Urethritis
Agrimony
Angelica
Cleavers
Cocklebur
Cota
Elder
Grindelia
Juniper
Mallow
Manzanita

Mormon Tea
Mullein
Pipsissewa
Plantain
Poplar
Pyrola
Storksbill
Uva Ursi
Willow
Yarrow
Yerba de la Negrita
Yerba Santa
Hematuria
Bugleweed
Raspberry
Red Root
Strawberry
Hyperacidity
Agrimony
Hyperalkalinity
Elder
Horsetail
Nettles
Poplar
Strawberry

Incontinence
Mullein
See DIURETIC

Kidney Stones
Asparagus
Chicory
Cleavers
Dandelion
Manzanita
Uva Ursi

Nephritis
Chicory
Cota

Dandelion
Milkweed
Pipsissewa
Pyrola
Uva Ursi

VASOCONSTRICTOR, SYSTEMIC
Avens
Bistort
Bugleweed
Cranesbill
Manzanita
Mistletoe
Nettles
Plantain
Red Root
Uva Ursi

VASODILATOR, SYSTEMIC
Bayberry
Motherwort
Oshá
Pennyroyal
Poleo
Spearmint

VOMITING/ NAUSEA
Alum Root
Angelica
Cow Parsnip
Cranesbill
Oshá
Pennyroyal
Poleo

WAX
Bayberry

WOOD CARVING
Manzanita

PLANT CLASSIFICATIONS

The sequence of families follows the traditional evolutionary system of Engler and Prantl.

I. Subkingdom PTERIDOPHYTA—
   Fern subkingdom
   POLYPODIACEAE (Polypody
   Fern family)
     Maidenhair Fern
   EQUISETACEAE (Horsetail family)
     Horsetail
II. Subkingdom SPERMATOPHYTA—
   Seed plants
   CLASS I—
   GYMNOSPERMAE—Cone-
   bearing plants
   PINACEAE (Pine family)
     Pine
   CYPRESSACEAE (Cypress family)
     Juniper
   GNETACEAE (Gnetum family)
     Mormon Tea
   CLASS II—ANGIOSPERMAE—
   Flowering plants
   A. Monocotyledons:
   LILIACEAE (Lily family)
     Agave

   Cañaigre
   Yellow Dock
   AMARANTHACEAE
   (Amaranth family)
     Amaranth
   NYCTAGINACEAE (Four-
   o'clock family)
     Maravilla
   RANUNCULACEAE (Butter-
   cup family)
     Baneberry
     Clematis
     Larkspur
     Marsh Marigold
     Peony
   BERBERIDACEAE (Barberry
   family)
     Oregon Grape
     Barberry
   LAURACEAE (Laurel family)
     California Bay
   PAPAVERACEAE (Poppy
   family)
     California Poppy
     Prickly Poppy

   Bush family)
     Burning Bush
   RHAMNACEAE (Buckthorn
   family)
     Coffee Berry
     Red Root
   MALVACEAE (Mallow family)
     Mallow
     Yerba de la Negrita
   STRECULIACEAE (Sterculia
   family)
     Fremontia
   HYPERICACEAE (Hypericum
   family)
     St. John's Wort
   ONAGRACEAE (Evening
   Primrose family)
     Evening Primrose
   UMBELLIFERAE (Parsley
   family)
     Angelica
     Cow Parsnip
     Oshá
   ERICACEAE (Heath family)

     Blue Curls
     Bugleweed
     Canip
     Horehound
     Motherwort
     Oregano de la Sierra
     Pennyroyal
     Poleo
     Sage
     Self Heal
     Skullcap
     Spearmint
   SOLANACEAE (Nightshade
   family)
     Jimson Weed
     Tobacco
   SCROPHULARIACEAE (Fig-
   wort family)
     Betony
     Figwort
     Mullein
     Penstemon
     Toadflax
   OROBANCHACEAE (Broom-

Amole Lily
Asparagus
False Solomon's Seal
Yucca
IRIDACEAE (Iris family)
  Blue Flag
ORCHIDACEAE (Orchid family)
  Rattlesnake Plantain
  Coral Root
B. Dicotyledons
SALICACEAE (Willow family)
  Willow
  Poplar
BETULACEAE (Birch family)
  Birch
FAGACEAE (Oak family)
  Oak
MORACEAE (Mulberry family)
  Hops
MYRICACEAE (Sweet-gale family)
  Bayberry
URTICACEAE (Nettle family)
  Nettle
LORANTHACEAE (Mistletoe family)
  Mistletoe
POLYGONACEAE (Buckwheat family)
  Bistort

FUMARIACEAE (Fumitory family)
  Corydalis
SAXIFRAGACEAE (Saxifrage family)
  Alum Root
ROSACEAE (Rose family)
  Agrimony
  Apache Plume
  Avens
  Mountain Mahogany
  Potentilla
  Raspberry
  Rose
  Strawberry
LEGUMINOSAE (Pea family)
  Alfalfa
  Licorice
  Red Clover
  Sweet Clover
GERANIACEAE (Geranium family)
  Cranesbill
  Storksbill
ZYGOPHYLLACEAE (Caltrop family)
  Contrayerba
RUTACEAE (Rue family)
  Hop Tree
CELASTRACEAE (Burning

Blueberry
Manzanita
Pipsissewa
Pyrola
Uva Ursi
GENTIANACEAE (Gentian family)
  Gentian
  Cebadilla
APOCYNACEAE (Dogbane family)
  Dogbane
ASCLEPIADACEAE (Milkweed family)
  Inmortal
  Pleurisy Root
  Milkweed
CONVOLVULACEAE (Morning-glory family)
  Dodder
HYDROPHYLLACEAE (Waterleaf family)
  Yerba Santa
BORAGINACEAE (Borage family)
  Hound's Tongue
VERBENACEAE (Verbena family)
  Blue Vervain
LABIATEAE (Mint family)

rape family)
  Broomrape
PLANTAGINACEAE (Plantain family)
  Plantain
RUBIACEAE (Madder family)
  Cleavers
CAPRIFOLIACEAE (Honey-suckle family)
  Elder
VALERIANACEAE (Valerian family)
  Valerian
LOBELIACEAE (Lobelia family)
  Lobelia
COMPOSITEAE (Sunflower family)
  Arnica
  Burdock
  Cachana
  Cat's Paw
  Chicory
  Cocklebur
  Coneflower
  Cota
  Dandelion
  Escoba de la Vibora
  Grindelia
  Wormwood
  Yarrow

REFERENCES AND FURTHER READING

BOTANY

ABRAMS, LEROY. *Illustrated Flora of the Pacific States*. 4 vols. Stanford University Press, Stanford, Calif., 1923–1960.

ARNBERGER, L. P., AND J. R. JANISH. *Flowers of the Southwest Mountains*. Southwest Parks and Monuments Assn., Globe, Ariz., 1962.

CRAIGHEAD, JOHN J. *A Field Guide to Rocky Mountain Wildflowers*. Houghton Mifflin Co., Boston, 1963.

DODGE, NATT. *100 Roadside Wildflowers of the Southwest Uplands*. Southwest Parks and Monuments Assn., Globe, Ariz., 1967.

————. *100 Desert Wild Wildflowers*. Southwest Parks and Monuments Assn., Globe, Ariz., 1963.

DODGE, NATT, AND J. R. JANISH. *Flowers of the Southwest Deserts*. Southwest Parks and Monuments Assn., Globe, Ariz., 1965.

HARRINGTON, H. D. *Manual of the Plants of Colorado*. Sage Books, Chicago, 1964.

HAUSMAN. *The Illustrated Encyclopedia of American Wildflowers*. Garden City Publishing Co., Garden City, N.Y., n.d.

JAEGER, EDMUND. *Desert Wild Flowers*. Stanford University Press, Stanford, Calif., 1956.

JEPSON, WILLIS. *Manual of the Flowering Plants of California*. University of California Press, Berkeley, 1960.

KEARNEY, THOMAS, AND ROBERT PEEBLES. *Arizona Flora*. University of California Press, Berkeley, 1964.

KELLY, GEORGE W. *A Guide to the Woody Plants of Colorado*. Pruitt Publishing Co., Boulder, Colo., 1970.

MUENSCHER, WALTER. *Poisonous Plants of the United States*. Collier Books, N.Y., 1961.

MUNZ, PHILIP A. *A California Flora*. University of California Press, Berkeley, 1968.

————. *A Flora of Southern California*. University of California Press, Berkeley, 1974.

————. *California Desert Wildflowers*. University of California Press, Berkeley, n.d.

————. *California Mountain Wildflowers*. University of California Press, Berkeley, 1963.

————. *California Spring Wildflowers*. University of California Press, Berkeley, n.d.

————. *Shore Wildflowers*. University of California Press, Berkeley, n.d.

NIEHAUS, T. F., AND C. L. RIPPER. *A Field Guide to Pacific States Wildflowers*. Houghton Mifflin Co., Boston, 1976.

PARSONS, MARY E. *The Wild Flowers of California*. Dover Publications, N.Y., n.d.

PATRAW, P. M., AND J. R. JANISH. *Flowers of the Southwest Mesas*. Southwest Parks and Monuments Assn., Globe, Ariz., 1973.

PECK. *A Manual of the Higher Plants of Oregon*. Binfords and Mort, Portland, n.d.

PRESTON, R. J. *Rocky Mountain Trees*. Dover Publications, N.Y., n.d.

RICKETT, HAROLD W. *Wild Flowers of the United States*. 6 vols. McGraw Hill Book Co., N.Y., 1966, 1973.
VINES, ROBERT A. *Trees, Shrubs, and Woody Vines of the Southwest*. University of Texas Press, Austin, 1960.
WEBER, WILLIAM A. *Rocky Mountain Flora*. Colorado Assn. University Press, Boulder, Colo., 1976.
ZIM, H. S., AND A. C. MARTIN. *Flowers*. Golden Press, N.Y., 1950.

HERBAL USE AND ETHNOBOTANY

BALLS, EDWARD K. *Early Uses of California Plants*. University of California Press, Berkeley, 1962.
CHAVEZ, TIBO J. *New Mexican Folklore of the Rio Abajo*. Bishop Printing Co., Portales, N.M., 1972.
CULBRETH, DAVID. *A Manual of Materia Medica and Pharmacology*. Health Research, Mokelumne Hill, Calif., 1927.
CURTIN, L. S. M. *Healing Herbs of the Upper Rio Grande*. Southwest Museum, Los Angeles, 1965.
FORD, KAREN. *Las Yerbas de la Gente*. Museum of Anthropology, University of Michigan, Ann Arbor, 1975.
GARDNER, J. L., ed. *Native Plants and Animals as Resources in Arid Lands of the Southwest*. Arizona State College, Flagstaff, 1965.
GILMORE, MELVIN. *Uses of Plants by the Indians of the Missouri River Region*. University of Nebraska Press, Lincoln, 1977.
GRIEVE, MAUD. *A Modern Herbal*. Dover Publications, N.Y., 1931.
HARPER, SHORE. *Prescriber and Clinical Repertory of Medicinal Herbs*. Health Science Press, Sussex, England, 1938.
HARRINGTON, H. D. *Edible Native Plants of the Rocky Mountains*. University of New Mexico Press, Albuquerque, 1967.
KIRK, DONALD. *Wild Edible Plants of the Western United States*. Naturegraph Publishers, Healdsburg, Calif., 1970.
LUST, JOHN. *The Herb Book*. Bantam Books, N.Y., 1974.
MEYER, JOSEPH. *The Herbalist*. Indiana Botanic Gardens, Hammond, n.d.
MILLSPAUGH, CHARLES. *American Medicinal Plants*. Dover Publications, N.Y., 1974.
MOORE, MICHAEL. *Los Remedios de la Gente*. Herbs Etc., Santa Fe, N.M., 1977.
OLIVER, J. H. *Proven Remedies*. Thorsons, Publishers, London, England, 1962.
POWELL, ERIC F. *The Modern Botanical Prescriber*. L. N. Fowler, London, England, 1965.
SMITH, F. P., AND G. A. STUART. *Chinese Medicinal Herbs*. Georgetown Press, San Francisco, 1973 reprint.
SWEET, MURIEL. *Common Edible and Useful Plants of the West*. Naturegraph Publishers, Healdsburg, Calif., 1962.
VOGEL, VIRGIL. *American Indian Medicine*. University of Oklahoma Press, Norman, 1970.
WEINER, MICHAEL A. *Earth Medicine—Earth Foods*. Collier Books, N.Y., 1972.
WREN, R. C. *Potter's New Cyclopedia of Botanical Drugs and Preparations*. Harper Row, N.Y., 1956.
A Barefoot Doctor's Manual. Running Press, Philadelphia, 1977.
Herbal Pharmacology in the People's Republic of China. National Academy of Sciences, Washington, D.C., 1975.

HOMEOPATHY

BOERICKE. *A Compend of the Principles of Homeopathy*. Health Research, Mokelumne Hill, Calif., n.d.
———. *Materia Medica with Repertory*. Boericke and Tafel, Philadelphia, 1927.
CLARKE, JOHN H. *A Clinical Repertory*. Health Science Press, Sussex, England, 1971.
———. *A Dictionary of Materia Medica*. 3 vols. Health Science Press, Sussex, England, 1962.
KENT, J. T. *Repertory of the Homeopathic Materia Medica*. Sett Dey and Co., Calcutta, India, 1961.
MHABJIA, K. C. *Master Key to Homeopathic Materia Medica*. National Homeo Laboratory, Calcutta, India, 1963.

MEDICAL AND PHARMACEUTICAL

GOODHART, R. S., AND M. E. SHILS. *Modern Nutrition in Health and Disease*. 5th ed. Lea and Febiger, Philadelphia, 1973.
MILLER, L. P., ed. *Phytochemistry,* Van Nostrand Rheinhold Co., N.Y., 1973.
ROBINSON, T. *The Organic Constituents of Higher Plants*. Burgess Publ., Minneapolis, 1967.
ROTHENBERG, R. E. *Medical Dictionary and Health Manual*. Signet Books, N.Y., 1975.
STEEN, EDWIN, AND ASHLEY MONTAGU. *Anatomy and Physiology*. 2 vols. Barnes and Noble, N.Y., 1959.
TREASE, G. E., AND W. C. EVANS. *A Textbook of Pharmacognosy*. 10th ed. Tindall and Cassell, London, England, 1972.
TYLER, VARRO E., LYNN R. BRADY, AND JAMES E. ROBBERS. *Pharmacognosy*. 7th ed. Lea & Febiger, Philadelphia, 1976.
TYLER, VARRO E., AND A. E. SCHWARTING. *Experimental Pharmacognosy*. 3rd ed. Burgess Publ., Minneapolis, 1962.
WALLIS, T. E. *Textbook of Pharmacognosy*. 5th ed. J and A Churchill, London, England, 1967.

Gray's Anatomy of the Human Body. 29th ed. Lea & Febiger, Philadelphia, 1973.
The Merck Index. 9th ed. Merck and Co., Rahway, N.J., 1976.
The Merck Manual. 13th ed. Merck and Co., Rahway, N.J., 1977.
Taber's Cyclopedic Medical Dictionary. 13th ed. F. A. Davis, Philadelphia, 1977.

WILDFLOWER HORTICULTURE

SPERKA, MARIE. *Growing Wildflowers*. Harper and Row, N.Y., 1973.
TAYLOR, K. S., AND S. F. HAMBLIN. *Handbook of Wildflower Cultivation*. Macmillan Publishing Co., N.Y., 1963.
TAYLOR, NORMAN. *Wildflower Gardening*. Van Nostrand, N.Y., 1955.

Gardening with Wild Flowers. Brooklyn Botanic Garden, Baltimore, 1974.
Propagation. Brooklyn Botanic Garden, Baltimore, 1974.

INDEX OF PLANT NAMES

Major entries are in capital letters, Latin generas in italics, and alternate plant names in roman (standard) type.